T0385439

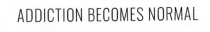
ADDICTION BECOMES NORMAL

SECTION SECOND

ADDICTION BECOMES NORMAL

On the Late-Modern
American Subject

JAEYOON PARK

The University of Chicago Press
Chicago and London

The University of Chicago Press, Chicago 60637
The University of Chicago Press, Ltd., London
Published 2024

Printed and bound by CPI Group (UK) Ltd, Croydon, CR0 4YY

33 32 31 30 29 28 27 26 25 24   1 2 3 4 5

ISBN-13: 978-0-226-82707-0 (cloth)
ISBN-13: 978-0-226-83276-0 (paper)
ISBN-13: 978-0-226-83275-3 (e-book)
DOI: https://doi.org/10.7208/chicago/9780226832753.001.0001

Library of Congress Cataloging-in-Publication Data

Names: Park, Jaeyoon, 1973– author.
Title: Addiction becomes normal : on the late-modern American subject /
    Jaeyoon Park.
Description: Chicago : The University of Chicago Press, 2024. | Includes
    bibliographical references and index.
Identifiers: LCCN 2023035295 | ISBN 9780226827070 (cloth) |
    ISBN 9780226832760 (paperback) | ISBN 9780226832753 (e-book)
Subjects: LCSH: Compulsive behavior. | Addicts. | Social norms.
Classification: LCC RC533.P267 2024 | DDC 616.85/227—dc23/
    eng/20230817
LC record available at https://lccn.loc.gov/2023035295

♾ This paper meets the requirements of ANSI/NISO Z39.48-1992
(Permanence of Paper).

Contents

Introduction

This book is about the normalization of addiction in the late-modern United States. Over the last forty years, a variety of developments in American science, politics, and culture have re-imagined addiction separately, yet in a common way. Increasingly, addiction is understood, no longer as an aberration of human experience, but as deeply normal, in a precise sense. Of course, it remains clear that addiction is not a modal condition, even as it is painfully common, among Americans. It remains clear, as well, that addiction is very rarely an easily lived state; more often, it entails deep devastation, sometimes even death. And yet today, leading voices across fields including medical science, public health, addiction treatment, and criminal justice insist that addiction is normal in the sense that, in its essence, addiction resembles our most ordinary attachments. They insist that a potential for addiction, or even a drive to addiction, is latent in all of us. And they insist that addiction is a predictable, even natural, response of the human being to what now so often surrounds us, namely, an ample and sure supply of potent thrills and pleasures. On such a view, the root of addiction is simply human nature, and the human is always, and from the start, an addict in waiting, if not in full. This book neither endorses nor refuses the view that addiction is normal, in these exact senses. Rather, it asks: Where and how has this view taken hold in our society? And what are the consequences of its rise for the way we imagine ourselves—what we are, how we live, and whether and how we can control our lives and ourselves?[1]

The normalization of addiction has not been a unitary or invariant process. I use the term *normalization* to designate a type of change that we can observe in a diversity of processes that have unfolded over the last forty years. Every case of normalization involves the production, or the mainstreaming, of a basic theory or figure of addiction that constructs it as analogous to and continuous with normal experience, within a given intellectual or professional domain. But this generic type of change has occurred differently in different domains. In medical science, it has occurred through the consolidation of the neurobehavioral figure of addiction as the dominant paradigm for scholarly research. In clinical practice, it has occurred through the establishment of the "dependence syndrome" model of addiction as the leading framework for diagnosis. In criminal justice, it has occurred through the invention of a new judicial instrument that identifies and treats addiction within the court. In recovery circles, it has occurred through the generalization and deep revision of twelve-step principles. And in the domains of treatment design and public policy, the normalization of addiction has taken still other forms.

Each of these developments warrants separate and detailed study, although that is not the project here. For their differences are deep and important. They vary, first of all, in historical kind: the consolidation of a dominant scientific paradigm is a very different process from the construction of a new judicial instrument, involving different types of actors, different motives, and different conditions of progress and failure. They vary, as well, in practical scope and effect. The neuroscientific paradigm has facilitated, and become bolstered by, an incredible range of experimental and observational studies; thus, it has had a huge effect on the scientific literature, and on what is cited as the science of addiction in public media, legal arguments, and state policy. Yet it has not yet yielded a novel and widely useful technique for treatment; hence, its power to change how institutions treat and respond to addiction has been weak.[2] By contrast, the judicial instrument of court-supervised treatment has had almost no effect, despite being grounded in its own explicit theory of addiction, on scholarly or public understandings of what addiction is. Yet the practice of court-supervised treatment has transformed how criminal justice handles addict-identified offenders in thousands of jurisdictions across the country. This points to another way in which the different cases of normalization vary: they pertain primarily to different populations, if not in principle, then in fact. The neuroscientific paradigm effectively normalizes addiction within medical research. But this matters only for those whose addictions are apprehended medically and described mainly in medical terms. In the United States, this means that the normalization of addiction by neuroscience pertains primarily to white addicts, and much less to Black or Hispanic addicts.[3] For its part, court-supervised treatment frames and handles the addictions of a much more racially heterogenous population.[4] But it makes no difference for those who live their addictions outside the criminal justice system.

Beneath these differences, however, there are also crucial commonalities across all the cases of normalization. These commonalities justify and focus the analytic approach taken here, which is to submit the normalization(s) of addiction to a more or less comprehensive study.

The first commonality is their temporal context. All the historical processes that we will be examining unfolded in a roughly bounded period, starting in the early 1980s and ending in the early 1990s. This is not to say that their temporalities are all exactly the same. To stay with our two featured examples: the rise of the neuroscientific paradigm of addiction could be traced back to preliminary research that was done, although not yet widely noticed, in the 1950s, whereas court-supervised treatment was a novel invention in the late 1980s.[5] And yet it was in the 1980s that both became fully established, mainstream, and prominent in their respective fields, and this general timing holds true for all the processes of normalization that this book studies.

Second, each case of normalization represents a promotion, and not just an appearance, of the view that addiction is normal in our time. That is, each normalizing development that we will study has coincided with the decline, in its domain, of earlier theories and practical models that constructed addiction as an abnormal form of experience. In addiction science, for instance, the last two decades of the twentieth century saw both the rise of the neuroscientific paradigm and the near-disappearance of theories that cast addiction as a symptom of psychopathology, which had been conventional in medical research for much of the twentieth century. Those decades surely did not see the replacement of disciplinary punishment by court-supervised treatment as the main state response to addiction, but such replacement did partially occur wherever drug courts emerged, and is often advocated in criminological discourse as an ideal. The rise of a new political rhetoric in the early 1990s, which casts addiction as an endemic public-health hazard, coincided with the decline of an alternative rhetoric that cast addiction as a threat to civilized society. And so forth. A coincidence of rise and decline is, of course, something less than a total paradigm shift. Still, it can constitute a trend—in this case, the promotion of normalizing theories of addiction over the alternative—and it demands our notice that the same trend has appeared in so many fields of reflection on addiction in late-modern American society.

The third commonality is that each process of normalization goes beyond a rethinking of addiction alone. In establishing the similarity of addiction to normal experience—or indeed their full homology, in some cases—the new theories of addiction that we will study all contribute to a more basic understanding of human nature and human experience. What is more, I will argue, all the normalizations of addiction converge on a certain way of figuring the human; despite their differences of idiom, motivation, and practical application, they all share a fundamental model or figure for understanding what the human creature is. Whether we are reading scientific theories of addictive desire, or analyzing the precepts of treatment by behavioral intervention, we will see the human figured as a creature whose personal dispositions are formed through a process of accretion, in whom the sheer repetition of certain acts, motivations, or desires over time leads these to become settled as an individual's characteristics or tendencies. Addiction is normal, we will see, because the human is *this* kind of creature, one whose lived desires and actions tend to harden and become persistent, even compulsive, through repetition. What is fascinating about this figure of the human is more than its enabling of the normalization of addiction. This is a figure of the human that allows us to represent the distinctive dispositions of a given person without making any stipulation of deep individuality—that is, without seeing one's dispositions as rooted in a personality, a psyche, or a soul. And it is a figure that, although unearthed in this book as the basis for all the normalizations of addiction, does not appear to have been made for only this purpose. Indeed, I will argue that it is a figure now often and widely used as a means of understanding the human in late-modern American culture and society.

All three commonalities justify a synthetic study of the normalization of addiction. But it is the third that most strongly motivates and shapes the character of this work. If the various normalizations of addiction were linked only by their temporal context and their manifestation of a roughly shared trend, then their significance would lie primarily in what they reveal about how American ideas about addiction have recently changed, and this book would be an entry in the history of ideas about addiction. But, as will soon become clear, this book is not really a work of intellectual history, in the ordinary sense. If it were, it would have two features which are in fact absent here. First, it would pay more attention to the limitations of the developments that we will be tracking within the domains where they have occurred. Clearly, no domain of science, policy, or medicine is ever a site of simple consensus, and indeed there are researchers who reject the neuroscience of addiction, even as they recognize its dominance, as well as treatment providers who use methods never advocated in contemporary professional journals. Second, a more conventionally historical work would develop much further the intellectual context within which all the normalizations of addiction have occurred. It would, for instance, feature analyses not just of contemporary medical and drug-policy literatures, but also of what we might call unofficial modes of thought about addiction: reflections on race, crime, poverty, and others in which addiction is constructed, in influential ways, but implicitly, often without even being named as addiction, instead figuring only as disorder, distress, or marginality. These two features would allow the study of normalization of addiction to situate this development within a fine-grained context of historical stasis and change, and also to illuminate that context as it exists today.

Of course, insofar as this book reveals one trend within contemporary thought about addiction, I do see it as advancing, without completing, that more historically oriented form of inquiry. A synthetic story of addiction's normalization has not yet been told. Yet crucially, it is also something else than a contribution to the history of ideas about addiction. It is primarily a work of cultural and political theory, and more specifically, a contribution to the genealogy of the late-modern American subject—or in other words, an inquiry into how the category of the human is distinctively and commonly constructed in our place and time. The wager of this work is that the normalizations of addiction not only influence how we now think about and treat the particular case of addiction, but refract and reveal a figure of the human that has become more and more common, in recent decades, as a way of imagining what we are in American society.

Because they are the framing terms of this work, I would like to develop a bit further the notions of *genealogy* and *the subject*. I invoke both with some hesitation, for both have become somewhat ossified over the years. Today, *genealogy* tends to refer, in cultural and political theory, to a particular method of research, and much effort has been devoted to specifying its procedures and validity. But here, I use the term in a more open-ended sense, as Foucault did in a 1983 interview. Asked to "describe the difference between archeology and genealogy from the point of view of historical methodology," Foucault complies, in part, by giving an account of "archeology" as a "material and methodological framework." But he then goes in a different direction, and describes "genealogy," not as a second method, but as a "motive and objective [*raison et objectif*]," or as a possible "purpose [*finalité*]" that might be pursued by any number of methods or styles of inquiry. Here, genealogy simply designates the objective, or purpose, of understanding the construction of "ourselves" and "our relation to ourselves and others . . . in our present." More concretely, it designates any work oriented toward shedding light on what "we" are in the present, and what allows or requires us to see "ourselves" in certain ways.[6]

But this is, of course, still ambiguous. What object is designated by "ourselves"? Here it helps to make a distinction between two possible referents: *subject* and *person*.[7] Whenever we refer to ourselves, we can do so in at least two ways. Asked to say who or what I am, I can reply first, in a Cartesian manner, and say "A man," or better, "A human." In other words, in referring to myself (or ourselves) I can describe *the kind of being* that I am, and develop the reference by stating the attributes that distinguish my kind of being. To do so is to refer to oneself as *subject*, that is, to invoke a general category that encompasses not just one's singular self but a range of similar beings. But second, one can also refer to oneself in a more particularizing way, and state not the kind of creature that one is but rather one's name or one's biography—what distinguishes this singular self from any other member of the category, human subject. One would then be referring to oneself as a *person*—not as *a* human, but rather as *this one*, this mind and body; not as "A man," but as René.

This is an elementary distinction, but it helps to make the object of genealogy clear. To be interested in the contemporary constitution of *ourselves* is plainly not to seek to know the life or makeup of any particular *person*. Rather, it is to wonder what constitutes the *subject* as a distinct category of being in our society. What particular attributes, tendencies, or capacities now define the category of the subject? What does it mean, now and precisely, to say that one is a *human*, and not another kind of being? And what determines that meaning?

Crucially, the *subject* and the *person* are not just conceptually distinct. They are formed through different processes. Who I am as a singular person is produced by the kinds of events and phenomena that tend to appear in memoirs, novels, and case histories. It is shaped by education and upbringing, engagements with intimate others, stasis or movement within social structures, and projects of self-direction and self-description. By contrast, the subject is constructed through the social production and dissemination of legitimate knowledge about the human. In Foucault's words, what it means to be human is constituted, first and foremost, by "discourses on the subject that are recognized institutionally or by consensus as true" within a given society.[8] Foucault's abstract proposition is easily made concrete. Our understanding of what we are, of how our minds, bodies, and selves are composed, is largely dependent on bodies of knowledge that are institutionalized or backed by expert consensus: scientific knowledge, medical theory, religious doctrine, philosophical reflection, and so forth. Thus, stipulating the target of genealogy as an understanding of the subject gives us an initial indication of what we need to study: bodies of knowledge that circulate truths about the nature or makeup of the human in our society.

To this rather simple point I now want to add a more speculative proposition. Clearly, the bodies of knowledge which are socially recognized as sources of insight into the subject are diverse and numerous. But our sense of what "we" are is not, I suggest, equally multiplicitous. Rather, in any given society, certain figures of the human are more prominent than others, more easily or widely accepted as a window onto the subject and its being. This prominence can arise in at least two different ways. First, it can result when a specific body of knowledge is actively promoted by an institution capable of undermining alternative sources of knowledge about the subject. Think, for instance, of the Church eliminating heretical discourses on the soul both by argument and by force. Second, the promotion of a certain figure of the human over others can result from the *convergence* of many different bodies of knowledge on a roughly similar understanding of the subject. In this case, a certain figure of the human gains influence, not by being uniquely enforced or imposed, but by gaining an unusually wide range of application and support—by appearing to be not the partisan production of one science, or tradition, or doctrine, but a common truth arrived at by so many different routes and confirmed by so many different intellectual sources.

That certain figures of the human wield an outsize influence on the definition of the subject in a given society, and that this outsize influence is rooted in the convergence of multiple bodies of knowledge—this proposition organized nearly all of Foucault's genealogical projects. Thus, for instance, in *Psychiatric Power* Foucault explains that his interest in nineteenth-century theories of madness is not fully intrinsic. Rather, what interests him above all is the "isotopy," or the isomorphism, between the figure of the human constructed by nineteenth-century psychiatry and that constructed by contemporaneous theories of worker discipline, education, and military training.[9] In all cases, Foucault shows, the human appears as the site of a deep essence or "core" that finds expression in the life and capabilities of the person who bears it—a "core" variously described, in different bodies of knowledge, as the psyche, as character, as intelligence, and as utility. Although these different bodies of knowledge were not directly conversant or linked with one another, they all served to support and advance a common figure of the human as a creature whose being is split between appearance and essence, whose life is the manifestation of a deep and determining core. Likewise, in *The History of Sexuality, Volume One*, Foucault is not interested in the modern sexual sciences entirely for themselves; he is interested in the construction of the Western subject as "a confessing animal," that is, as a creature with a hidden identity that can be revealed in, and extracted from, self-referential language. As is well known, this is a construction that Foucault finds developed and bolstered not only in the modern sexual sciences, but also in the philosophical, religious, and criminological theories that arose just before or alongside them.[10]

The thesis that certain figures of the human have an outsize importance in any given society, and that this importance rests on a convergence of diverse knowledges, also serves as the organizing premise of the present attempt at genealogy. In theorizing the normalization of addiction, I am interested above all in the larger figure of the human that appears across all the different normalizing theories, models, and frameworks for addiction that we will analyze. For once we reveal this larger figure of the human, we will find that it is a figure that is featured across a wide range of sites, far beyond the domains of thought about addiction, in late-modern American society. Like the figure of the human as the site of an essential "core" that Foucault discovered in so many sciences and other bodies of knowledge about the subject in nineteenth-century Western societies, the figure of the human as a site of dispositional accretion through repeated experience has a wide variety of instantiations and appearances in our time. It appears as the basis for, and implication of, the normalization of addiction. But, as we will see, it appears as well, albeit differently, in the model of the psyche advanced by what is now the dominant mode of psychotherapy in the United States, namely, cognitive behavior therapy. It appears in new and increasingly popular methods of human evaluation and assessment, such as rating, self-tracking, and the construction of digital profiles. It appears in the ubiquitous language and paradigm of wellness, now nearly a synonym for self-care and health. These are, at least, the appearances that we will explicitly analyze in the course of this inquiry; likely, the list could long go on.

Thus, the figure of the human revealed by the normalization of addiction is important for a genealogy of the late-modern American subject insofar as it is a recurrent, multiply supported, and thus powerfully promoted construction of ourselves in our time. This figure is important for our genealogy in a second way. Foucault was right, I think, to see the figure of the human as the site of a "core" or "essence" as ubiquitous throughout modern Western societies. His revelation of this figure has, of course, illuminated the structure and effect of numerous modern forms of knowledge about the subject: not only nineteenth-century knowledges, but also twentieth-century versions of psychiatry, psychology, criminology, philosophy, and more. Yet one question that his work now raises is whether that figure of the human as the site of an essence remains ubiquitous, live, and influential in our own time, half a century after Foucault conducted his studies. Of course, the scope of the current project will not allow us to demonstrate the full absence of any particular figure of the human in our society. What we will find, however, is that in almost every case the figure of the human that is at the center of the present study—that is, the figure of the human as *accretion*—is a direct, and often quite explicit, challenge to the figure of ourselves as bearers of cores. The normalization of addiction very often proceeds as a direct repudiation of the idea that compulsive desire or conduct reflects an underlying spirit, psyche, or soul. The reimagination of psychic experience achieved by cognitive behavior therapy is a challenge to the psychoanalytic construction of experience as the surface expression of a deep and stable personal unconscious. The promotion of wellness is premised on a repudiation of the idea that how we live, and what we do, is the manifestation of an inner will, or any other kind of individual sovereign force. In short, the figure of the human as accretion appears, in each case, as a displacement of, and not just a neutral alternative to, the figure of ourselves as sites of expression for a personal essence. Again, this does not show that the figure of essence has completely disappeared around us. But it may show that ours is a society in which the figure of essence is becoming less influential, and less widely supported. Or at least, that ours is a society in which challenges to the figure of essence have emerged, alongside it, as a crucial influence on the definition of the subject. Either way, we would have an important genealogical insight, a sense not just of what the late-modern American subject increasingly is, but also of what it may now be less, if not no longer.

Genealogy cannot but be speculative, but it is also gray, as Foucault famously put it.[11] I have been open about the assumptions that organize this project, but the core arguments of the book are based on empirical analysis. That the normalizations of addiction have occurred, that they forward a larger figure of the human, and that this figure of the human is echoed well outside the ambit of thought about addiction in late-modern US society and culture— these are claims to be proved through close readings of primary documents in the coming chapters. That this figure is, by virtue of its recurrence and its departure from the figure of essence, an especially important constituent of the subject in our time is a more speculative assertion, but one that will draw force, if not full confirmation, from the more conventionally grounded claims. It will also draw force, to the extent that it is true, from its capacity to resonate with readers' experiences. If I am right that the figure of accretion is now a significant construction of the subject, then it will be familiar to readers who have never examined the bodies of knowledge from which this book unearths that figure in a deep and deliberate way. One aim of this book is precisely to attune us to the fact that this figure has become familiar to us, without our having sought it out, and in spite of its recency as well as its lingering strangeness.

More modestly, this book aims, first, to consolidate the normalization of addiction as a frame for interpreting a wide range of recent developments in addiction theory and practice, and second, to insist that such an interpretation casts important light on the constitution of the late-modern American subject. To do this, all of the chapters move between two registers. Much of my argument consists in detailed analyses of texts drawn from the fields of addiction science, public health, criminal justice, mutual help, and so forth, through which I hope to render the sense and reality of normalization firmly grounded and clear. At the same time, I draw these historical texts into more philosophical discussions, asking what they imply about the nature and life of the human, and how they recast and invent crucial aspects of the category of the subject. The progression of the book as a whole is an expansion of focus. The first chapters are mostly concerned with tracing and developing the normalizations of addiction, whereas later chapters spend more time examining the concordances between normalizing theories of addiction and other recent transformations of American society and culture. For most of the book I stay close to the language of the texts that I am reading, while also laying ground for a more comprehensive theorization of the figure of the human that they build. In other words, throughout the work I try to show that the figure of accretion emerges, variously but persistently, in all the texts that I am reading. But only at the end of the book will I name this figure in this way, for doing so too early would risk obscuring the really specific ways in which the figure of accretion takes shape.

Having set forth the project's aim and scope, I now turn to a more detailed outline of its chapters.

Chapter 1, "The Normalization of Addiction," establishes the precise meaning and key instances of the phenomenon that forms the basis for this book. *Normalization,* as I use the term in this book, does not essentially refer to an increased cultural acceptance of addiction, or to a greater recognition that morally and psychologically normal people can suffer addiction, too—although both are certainly possible effects of normalization. Rather, it refers to the emergence or novel acceptance of the idea that *addiction itself is normal,* in the sense that addictive craving and compulsion are simply strong versions of normal (healthy, quotidian) desire and conduct, not aberrant ways of being. The chapter clarifies this sense of normalization, and begins sketching its historical reality, by closely analyzing what I consider the four crucial cases of normalization in the late twentieth century. In the domain of laboratory science, we will chart the ascendance of the neurobehavioral model of addiction as a dominant paradigm; in clinical diagnostics, we will see the dissolution of addiction and its recasting as a "syndrome" in the *Diagnostic and Statistical Manual of Mental Disorders* and the *International Classification of Diseases*; in criminal justice, we will chart the invention and steady dissemination of the new technique of court-supervised treatment; in the policy sphere, we will see the mainstreaming of a new rhetorical frame for drug and addiction crises. In different ways, all these transformations reject an earlier construction of addiction, within their domain, as manifesting an abnormal desire, pleasure, or mode of conduct, and construct addiction instead as an extension or intensification of normal experience. The four cases examined in this chapter provide a clear template of normalization, but also an indication of the range and extent of normalizing processes, which in the last two decades of the twentieth century emerged in a variety of fields with considerable social influence and reach.

The subsequent chapters continue to develop our sense of the meaning and reality of the normalization of addiction by analyzing further cases, but take up a second task, as well. Chapter 2, "The Power of Behavioral Interventions," argues that the rise of behavioral interventions as the most common modality of addiction *treatment* over the last thirty years (this is not to say that they are the most common *social response* to addiction) constitutes another crucial instance of normalization in recent American history. It then reads this development, not just as a rethinking of how addiction can most effectively be treated, but as a new understanding of what the subject is, and how its behavior can be controlled. Placing behavioral interventions in contrast to a mode of treatment that remained widely popular until the end of the twentieth century—the therapeutic community—I show that behavioral interventions constitute what recent scholars have termed a *post-disciplinary* approach to figuring and changing subjective conduct. That is, they constitute an approach to figuring and changing the acting subject which is distinguished (1) by its elision of the personality or character of the subject; (2) by a reluctance to exercise direct control over the subject; and (3) by a faith in the capacity of gentle and unforced exposures of the subject to new rewards to alter the inner motives and outward life of that subject. This reimagination of the subject, the chapter shows, accompanies the normalization of addiction in the field of treatment; but it is also instanced elsewhere in contemporary US society, as various cultural and political theorists have shown in their analyses of neoliberalism, digital profiling, and penal rationality. In making this dual argument, the chapter raises the possibility that the normalization of addiction contributes to and reflects a broader construction of the subject under way in our time.

Chapter 3, "Measuring Our Desire," raises that possibility again, but by a different route. It begins by analyzing the neuroscientific theory of incentive-salience attribution, which now serves as the leading explanation of what addictive craving is, and how it develops, in venues ranging from medical textbooks on addiction to TV documentaries on the science and experience of addiction. I show that this theory, as originally presented, was aimed at revising the Freudian and Skinnerian views of desire that informed much of the psychological work on addiction in the twentieth century, and that the theory achieved this revision by offering a new basic account of human desire. In this account, desire is naturally and always *inaugurated by a stimulating object*, not emanated from the subject's interior; *compounded by repeated cases of stimulation*, rather than formed by stable personal drives or ideas; and *properly registered as a metric quantity*, not as a linguistic or symbolically organized entity. This reimagination of desire is a crucial aspect of the scientific normalization of addiction; it reduces the difference between addictive craving and normal desire to magnitude or intensity, and enables the scientific view of craving as desire's "quantitative maximum." But here again, as in the previous chapter, the case of normalization being examined also bears a larger significance. I argue that the recasting of desire as a metric quantity, produced through the stimulation of the self by an object, is not just an achievement of recent addiction science. It is a transformation achieved, or at least furthered, as well, by a range of other recent developments in US society, including the rise of cognitive behavior therapy, the popularization of self-tracking, and the spread of ratings as measures of value and desirability. Alongside these other developments, the normalization of craving will appear as one of several means for a more general reconceptualization of the subject's desire in our time: precisely not as a secret to be confessed, as Foucault described the construction of desire most ubiquitous in Western modernity, but as a kind of amassed quantity, built up in the subject by the powerful stimulation of objects.

The fourth and last main chapter, "Reframing the Self," examines what I call the mode of self-relation promoted by a range of recent texts on addictive compulsion. Reading public-health documents, psychological theory, and twelve-step manuals, I show that addictive compulsion is today often explained by reference to a more general understanding of human conduct. The texts that I examine all argue that in order to understand compulsion, we first need to see our conduct in a precise way, namely, as the product of a host of influences and forces impinging upon the subject, and competing with one another to determine what the subject will do. The crucial point, in this view, is not that the subject's conduct is strictly determined. It is that no single force ever determines the subject's conduct alone, and that conduct is always the outcome of the balance or sum of forces weighing on the subject. These forces include legal proscriptions, social pressures, and biological drives, as well as conscious intention—the last is always present, and active, as a force contending to determine the act of the subject, but always in contention, always only as *one* ingredient in the production of conduct. This general understanding of conduct clarifies addictive compulsion: no longer the result of an impaired capacity for sovereign self-direction (there is no such capacity), compulsion is simply a condition in which the single force of conscious intention is overpowered by, and at odds with, what the balance of forces acting on the subject press one to do. This general understanding of conduct does something more. It opens up a new and entire perspective on the subject's self-relation, that is, on how the subject can and should seek to influence its life and its conduct. In this perspective, we control ourselves, not by hardening our wills or by purifying our intentions, but by adjusting the array of powers to which we are persistently exposed. We move away from certain influences and into the arms of others; we numb ourselves to certain attractions and bind ourselves to better ones. In elaborating this mode of self-relation promoted by recent texts on addictive compulsion, we will find ourselves using an idiom most thoroughly developed in the recently popularized discourse of *wellness*. Drawing the writings on compulsion and the foundational texts on wellness together, this chapter casts both as engaged in a common and ongoing project of recasting the subject's relation to itself, and capacity for self-direction, in our society.

The book concludes with an effort to synthesize and name the imagination of ourselves—the subject—that the main chapters illuminate in partial ways. To do this, the conclusion stages a contrast between the subject for whom addiction is a permutation of normal desire and conduct and what Foucault theorized as the dominant figure of the subject in modern Western societies. Across his major works, Foucault showed that many of the most influential forms of science and politics in the modern West figured the subject, in one way or another, as constituted around and by an *essence* which is expressed in the subject's manifest life and body. Modern sexual science, for instance, cast sexual desire and actions as expressions of psychic structure, or of "sexuality"; likewise, modern criminology was organized by an understanding of criminal "instinct" as lying beneath and causing criminal deeds. Foucault's theorization of the modern subject as a creature of essence will serve us as a model of what is challenged and remade through the normalization of addiction. Each of the theories and practices studied in this book's main chapters is more than an innovation; each claims to be an *advance* on an older theory or practice that posits an essence behind the subject in explaining or treating addiction. Thus, behavioral interventions promise to replace punitive approaches to therapy which posit an immature psyche, or primitive character, behind the manifest symptoms of addiction. The dependence-syndrome theory that now frames the *DSM* criteria for addiction diagnosis was designed to shatter and retire the idea that addiction can be traced to a single etiology or source in the patient. What is more, I argue that, at a general level, the theories and practices that this book gathers under the rubric of addiction's normalization all challenge the figure of essence in a broadly uniform way. They cast the subject's typical desires and behaviors, not as expressions of a stable, underlying essence or core—a psyche, a character, or a soul—but rather as hardened accretions built up through the accumulation and repetition of similar experiences. My desire is formed, not in the crucible of my soul, but in the course of my lived history, as I enjoy the same object again and again, until that object becomes special, reliable, and familiar, and thus an object of steady desire for me. Likewise my habits, and my behavioral tendencies, do not express a personal project or moral compass; they simply extend a series, as it were, or continue a pattern established only by my performance of a certain act many times in the past, regardless of whether that act was first chosen by or forcibly imposed on me. Who I am is constituted, in this vision, as the accretion of what I have desired, done, and experienced; such accretion is my life and my character, my past and my identity.

To the extent that this vision of the subject's constitution contrasts with what Foucault theorized as the common subject of Western modernity, and to the extent that it finds support not only in the normalizations of addiction, but in the broader range of theories and practices studied in this book, the subject of accretion may well be considered a crucial figure for the late-modern American subject—a figure imagined in many ways, and increasingly familiar and common, in our society. To be sure, it is not the only figure for us circulating in our day, and yet it may serve as one important answer to what Foucault gave us as the genealogical question: the question of what it means to be human—what the category *human* designates—here and now, in our social place and time. The book ends with ambivalence about what it finds: on the one hand, with relief, in the thought of being more and more surrounded by a figure that refuses to read our desires or our lives as signs of flaws and failures deep inside us; on the other, with some worry, about another set of means in the late-modern world for imagining ourselves as creatures without soul, without essence.

ONE

The Normalization
of Addiction

It is one common practice, in both scholarly and popular discourse, to represent thinking about addiction in America as an activity, or process, of *abjection*.[1] Consider this fable, written by Eve
Kosofsky Sedgwick in 1993. "Once upon a time," she tells us, "back
in the old country, some people sometimes took opium." These
nameless folk did so, presumably, for a wide variety of reasons,
but these reasons were not closely regarded, let alone recorded. In
short, neither drug use nor its motives were topics of organized
knowledge. Drug use was "a behavior among other behaviors," and
it was enough to leave it at that. But then, in "the late nineteenth
century," a new era opened—"something changed"—and there
emerged a concerted effort to produce knowledge about addiction
in the fields of medicine and law. Two things resulted from this
effort. First, drug use was now sharply distinguished as a form of
behavior, and those who engaged in drug use were likewise differ-
entiated, cast as deeply different, from other humans. In Sedgwick's words, "Under the taxonomic pressures of a newly rami-
fied and pervasive medical-juridical authority," "what had been a
question of acts crystallized into a question of identity." There was
"a taxonomic reframing of the drug user as an addict," or a construction of the addict as a distinct human category. Second, and
simultaneously, the addict was constructed as a degraded type of
human, as a fallen and not neutrally unique sort of creature. The

addict was understood, both in medicine and in law, as someone who had diverged from the normal life of the human through "a narrative of inexorable decline and fatality," a collapse of morals, mind, or body. In short, the emergence of organized knowledge about addiction involved the construction of "a newly pathologized addict identity," an identity whose assumption casts the one who bears it as deviant and in need of correction: to be an addict was to be "the proper object of compulsory institutional disciplines, legal and medical." Since the late nineteenth century, Sedgwick continues, the making of knowledge about addiction has remained a "taxonomic frenzy," a roving and restless quest to find, construct, and tar as deviant "the next pathologized personage," whether at the site of drug use, or at that of any other potentially addictive human activity.[2]

The language of Sedgwick's story makes its status as fable clear. And yet the narrative form it exemplifies is often used for more realistic representations. This narrative form, which is likely familiar to most readers, casts knowledge about addiction as a means of *pathologization*, or better, *abjection*. (Represented, after all, is not just the identification of a disease, but the casting of the disease as an abject condition, and related, the denigration of those who bear the disease.) In other words, it casts the process of knowing or producing knowledge about addiction as a procedure in which a certain group of people (drug users, gamblers, consumers) is conceptually cordoned off from all other human beings; named with a distinct label or identity category (drug addict, gambling addict, shopping addict); and finally negatively evaluated as lacking, in some essential respect, compared to those who live without that label or category. Sedgwick and other cultural theorists have used this narrative form to represent the general production of knowledge about addiction in Western societies; *all* knowledge about addiction, in their narratives, involves the construction of addiction and the addict as abject categories. But it can also be used to describe a particular body of knowledge about addiction, such as a specific scientific theory, or media coverage of a specific addiction outbreak. The narrative form of abjection can also capture what we might call quotidian productions of knowledge about addiction, such as the self-description of an addict-identified person to their friends, or the discovery and description of an adolescent's addiction by their parents. The narrative form of abjection has many possible applications.

And indeed, the narrative form of abjection throws light on many historical realities. As we will see, for instance, the scientific theories of addiction that rose to national prominence just after the time period featured in Sedgwick's story—that is, in the 1920s and 1930s—constructed addiction as a sign of deep psychopathology. Although anyone might become physiologically dependent on certain drugs, truly compulsive drug use revealed the addict's inability to deal with the stresses of social existence in any other way, consequent to abnormal development of psyche and personality. Addiction thus indexed psychic disorder, and the addict was abject, in the sense of being figured as distinct, broken, and deviant. Or consider the ready example of how addicts were known in the political rhetoric and news media of the War on Drugs period. The words of William Bennett leap to mind: "Drugs destroy the natural sentiments and duties that constitute our human nature and make our social life possible." Hence Bennett equated being "an addict" with being "on the street, in the gutter, a burnt-out case." Accordingly, Bennett promoted the work of addiction recovery programs, developed in the 1970s and 1980s, that were modeled on "two institutions: the military for teaching discipline and the church for nourishing the soul."[3] Here again, we encounter knowledge that constructs the addict as an abject identity: as a creature fallen from human nature, without discipline, wrecked in soul. And then there are, of course, the many outright hostile forms of knowledge, cultural and popular, for which abjection is a driving purpose and not just a narrative form: the construction of stories, images, and language about the homeless junkie, or the crack mother—deviations not just from the human, but also from gender, class, and racial norms.

For all its uses, however, there are historical realities that the narrative form of abjection obscures. In fact, this chapter argues that some of the most important developments in our recent history concerning how addiction is known in the United States are legible only if we set aside the narrative form of abjection in favor of another, which is its inverse. This is the narrative form of *nor-*

malization. One trend of the last forty years, I will show, has been the rise to prominence, across a variety of influential domains of thought about addiction (including science, medicine, and criminal justice), of theories, models, and other means of understanding addiction that cast it precisely *not* as a condition belonging to an abject few, who are different in essence from all other human beings, and *instead* as a possible development and natural tendency in every human subject. In short, one trend of our time (not the only trend, but a crucial one no less) has been the construction of addiction and the addict as normal across a variety of domains in American society, or what I call the *normalization of addiction.* Here, normalization does not mean the forced assimilation of unruly behaviors to the norm; nor does it refer to an increasing moral or cultural acceptance of addiction. Rather, the process of normalization should be understood as the contrary of abjection: it is a process through which addiction is *analogized to* or constructed as *continuous with* normal experience, and through which the addict is cast as a normal subject, not an exceptional type of being.

If normalization is conceptually contrary to abjection, this does not mean that the rise of normalization as a trend in our recent history implies the decline or cessation of abjection in our time. The claim here is only that within and across the domains of knowledge that we will be studying, normalization has emerged as a distinct and major trend. Beyond these domains, and at their margins, abjection surely still proceeds in various ways. The narrative of this chapter neither denies nor inspects the coexistence of normalization and abjection as trends in American thought about addiction. Instead, it focuses on revealing just how widely and effectively the normalization of addiction is occurring in late-modern American society. It is a striking fact of our culture and our time that so many of our most influential sources of knowledge about addiction—scientific theories, diagnostic manuals, judicial frameworks, public policy—have the effect of normalizing addiction, of rendering it as a normal condition, and of casting the addict as a figure that encompasses or awaits us all. Only in the past forty years, I will argue, has normalization become a dominant and mainstream process within each of the four domains that this chapter studies. In tracing how this has happened across a range of social spheres in our recent history, this chapter proposes normalization as *one* crucial means of characterizing how addiction is thought and known in our society.

The ramifications and cultural significance of the fact that the normalization of addiction has emerged as a trend in late-modern American society will be the sustained topic of chapters to come, which ask the question of what the emergence of normalization as a contemporary trend reveals about how human desire, will, and selfhood are more generally imagined and figured in our cultural place and time. In this chapter, our task is to firmly establish the precise shape and scope of the trend of normalization. To do this, I examine what I consider the four most important recent instances of this trend: the rise to prominence of behavioral and neuroscientific paradigms of addiction in scientific research in the course of the 1980s; the development of a new diagnostic framework for addiction in the leading psychiatric manuals, also in the 1980s; the invention of a new judicial theory and framework for addressing addiction within the criminal justice system in the late 1980s and early 1990s; and the promotion of a new national political rhetoric for framing drug use and addiction starting in the early 1990s. In charting each of these cases in turn, my aim is to show how despite their patent differences, all instantiate a general pattern, and unfold within a bounded period. Beginning in the final decades of the twentieth century, and extending into our own time, each of the developments to be traced effectively displaces a previously influential form of knowledge that constructed addiction and the addict as deviant or abnormal, and yields a new type of knowledge—a new theory, or model, or terminology—that recasts addiction and the addict as akin to, or even isomorphic with, normal desire, conduct, and being. Our interest is both in how these developments instantiate the pattern of normalization and in their individual histories; we must apprehend both if normalization is to be viewed not merely as a narrative form, but as the real structure of the historical developments that form the basis of this book.

Scientific Research

The field of addiction science is vast and variegated, and it forwards no theses as a whole. And yet, there are historical changes that have ramifications throughout the field, and it is one such change that we are tracking here. This is the rise of behavioral research and neuroscience as the mainstream approaches to addiction science in the last quarter of the twentieth century. Several historians of addiction, as well as internal accounts of the field, have effectively charted this rise, showing how federal funding streams for addiction research increasingly ran to those using behavioral and neuroscientific approaches starting in the late 1970s, and how the leaders of institutions such as the National Institute on Drug Abuse were increasingly drawn from the ranks of behavioral researchers and neuroscientists.[4] Today in the public sphere, when recent advances in addiction science are touted, it is often the results of neuroscience alone that are featured.[5] Thus, the implications of behavioral and neuroscientific research have an outsize influence on both the real output and the public reception of the addiction-science field.

Our task is not to retrace the promotion of behavioral and neuroscientific approaches to the mainstream of addiction science. Rather, it is to illuminate a particular consequence of this promotion. As I will show, one of the distinctive features of the behavioral and neuroscientific approaches is their acceptance and confirmation of the idea that the addict's attachment to drugs is identical in kind with the attachment of any subject to any object, including those that bind us to basic and vital objects such as food, sex, and love. In other words, the notion that addictive and nonaddictive attachments are essentially similar, although different in magnitude, recurs as a conclusion of behavioral and neuroscientific research. Hence, as these approaches have moved to the center of the addiction-science field in our time, so too has the notion that addiction is an extension of normal attachment gained the status of a mainstream truth forwarded by the leading research on addiction in late-modern American society. Such is the first historical process for us to consider: the homologization of addictive and nonaddictive attachments in the mainstream of contemporary addiction research.

To grasp the significance of this development, we require some historical background. It would be too strong, of course, to say that the theorization of a homology between addictive and nonaddictive attachments was never anticipated in addiction research prior to the late-twentieth century. Yet we can show that just the opposite premise was a central feature in many influential theories of addiction throughout the mid-twentieth century. That is, the scholars who now figure most prominently in histories of addiction science almost invariably conceived addiction as an abnormal modality of attachment to an object. This is not to say that these scholars conceived addiction as immoral or worthy of condemnation; most often, they saw it as a site for therapeutic intervention and care. It is rather to say that many of the most influential theorists of addiction in the mid-twentieth century saw addiction as *essentially dissimilar* from the normal, unproblematic relations between most subjects and what they consume. Most saw addiction, further, as the sign of a *subjective difference* between addicts and nonaddicts, as if an abnormal relation to objects were rooted in an unusually formed psyche, consciousness, or soul.

Consider, for instance, the views of the psychiatrist Lawrence Kolb, founding director of the US government's major prison-hospital for addicts, and by all accounts the most influential theorist of addiction in the mid-twentieth century. Kolb's influence was twofold. First, he was responsible for most widely promulgating the "psychopathy theory" of addiction, which held that addictive cravings symptomatize a basic defect of character or personality. He was hardly alone in articulating the view, but, as the historian David Courtwright puts it, Kolb most powerfully "systematized and popularized" the psychopathy theory and rendered it "a veritable cliché in the addiction literature" through a series of seminal articles.[6] Kolb's influence also went beyond the field of addiction research. As the historian Caroline Acker has shown, "Kolb's views became the basis for constructing the addict as social deviant" in policy circles, and justified "the prevailing enforcement policy that called for arrest and imprisonment for possession of opiates," despite Kolb's own opposition to such policies.[7] The second means of Kolb's influence was his design of a typological system that classed addicts according to "the degree of psychopathology [they] exhibited." According to the historian Nancy Campbell, this system, known as the K-classification scheme, was "used to categorize addicts for decades" in both clinical practice and research.[8] Let us examine Kolb's classification scheme and basic theory in turn.

There are two ways of reading Kolb's classification scheme. On the first reading, the scheme covers *five* categories of addicts. "Class I" includes "mentally healthy persons who had become addicted accidentally or necessarily through the use of narcotic drugs for the treatment of an illness." Each of the remaining Classes, II–V, identifies an addict group according to the "psychiatric disturbance" that causes the addiction: psychoneurosis (II), character disorder (III), personality disorder (IV), sociopathic personality (V). On this reading, then, addicts appear to fall into two broad categories: "mentally healthy," on one hand, and "psychiatrically disturbed," on the other.[9] Campbell, for instance, adopts this reading when she summarizes Kolb's scheme as divided into "two primary categories," the "accidentally addicted . . . but otherwise normal" and "those predisposed by psychopathology to the 'vicious' pleasures . . . of narcotic drugs."[10]

But there is another way of reading Kolb's classification, which finds that there are really only *four* categories of addicts, namely, the disturbed classes. This appears to have been the more common reading among Kolb's contemporaries. Courtwright, for instance, argues that one major effect of Kolb's growing influence in the 1930s and beyond was that "the view that addicts were normal persons addicted accidentally was all but abandoned" in the field.[11] In fact, Kolb included *and* excluded such "normal" addicts from his scheme. They were included, under Class I, but also identified as "the exception among the five classes." Moreover, Kolb often excluded Class I addicts from general discussions of the scheme. Thus, he presented the scheme as establishing that to "the question whether drug addicts are recruited from the ranks of the mentally ill," "the answer is affirmative."[12] All addicts, then, are really drawn from Classes II to V.

One reason for Kolb's exclusion of Class I addicts from the system proper was historical. He believed that the passage of the Harrison Narcotic Act in 1914, which restricted the ability of most physicians to dispense opiates, would eliminate the phenomenon of "accidental" addictions. In fact, all the cases of Class I addiction that he had tallied "had originated prior to 1915, the year when the Harrison Narcotic Law became effective."[13] But there was also a deeper reason for the exception, rooted in theory. Kolb believed that a truly compulsive addiction to drugs, as opposed to mere physical dependence, could not be caused by prescribed drug use alone. Rather, he held that the compulsiveness characteristic of a genuine addiction revealed the presence of a special kind of *pleasure* in the addict's relationship to the drug, one that had its conditions in the psychic constitution of the addict. In a paper published shortly after his introduction of the classification scheme, Kolb explained that in order to understand addiction,

> one must distinguish between the pleasure that is merely a reflex following relief from anxiety and pain and the pleasure which an individual experiences when he is lifted above his usual emotional plane. The reflex from relief of conditions that are temporary or accidental may be termed negative pleasure. Relief from conditions that are more or less permanent or fundamental may be termed positive pleasure.[14]

He continues: "normal as well as abnormal persons receive negative pleasure" from the use of drugs. For anyone, that is, drugs produce pleasure by relieving *temporary* conditions like acute bodily pains, or even heartache and grief. Yet "rarely, if ever, does anyone except the psychopath and the neurotic experience positive pleasure."[15] This is because only abnormal persons, such as these, suffer emotional distress and suffering as a *permanent* and *fundamental* condition. Only "the abnormal man with feelings of inferiority and a highly sensitive or poorly organized nervous system" experiences all of life as a stressor and disappointment, lacking the inner capacities that would allow him to fit in comfortably and find acceptance as a normal member of society. Thus, only the abnormal man "is always striving for an emotional something just out of his normal reach," always yearning for a basic sense of calm and satisfaction ever precluded by his sense of inner turmoil and insufficiency. "Alcohol or drugs brings it [the 'emotional something' sought by the abnormal person] within his normal range and gives him the satisfaction that he does not know how to obtain in any other way." For the abnormal person, in short, the drug brings not just acute relief, but the positive pleasure of freedom from permanent inner pain. This is why addicts cannot give up the objects of their addiction, even at the cost of a prison sentence, waning health, or social condemnation. What is the pain of confinement or bodily deterioration, after all, next to the feelings of deep disturbance and misfit that color every moment of an abnormal person's existence? "The causes of addiction and relapse are fundamentally the same," Kolb insisted; they are to be "found in the addict's faulty mental make-up" and what this leads them to seek: "the pleasurable sense of relief from the realities of life that normal persons do not receive [from drug use] because life is no special burden to them."[16]

Thus, at the heart of Kolb's theory and classificatory scheme was the idea that addiction constitutes a unique relationship between subject and object, and that the compulsiveness of an addiction represents something more than a quantitative increase of ordinary motivation. And as his theory and schema spread, so too did this premise of a generic difference between addictive and nonaddictive attachments. And yet the prevalence of this basic premise exceeded the ambit of Kolb's influence in mid-twentieth-century addiction research. Nancy Campbell has shown that through the 1950s, psychoanalysis was a central disciplinary source for addiction research in the United States.[17] It is thus significant that in the work of Sandor Rado, whom Campbell identifies as "the most influential psychoanalyst working in the addictions field" in his time, we find an alternative to Kolb's theory of addiction that promotes, in its own way, the notion that addictive attachments essentially differ from ordinary subject-object relations.[18] Rado rejected the view of psychiatrists like Kolb, which he criticized as too vague in its tracing of addiction to an abnormal constitution. He sought to explain the psycho*dynamics* by which drug use becomes an addiction, and argued that addiction must be understood as part of a distinctive "regime" of emotional regulation. Rado posited that there is "a group of human beings who respond to frustrations in life with a special type of emotional alteration," in which the psyche reacts to frustrations by developing a general sense of depression. This allows the subject to relieve distress, not by working through particular feelings, but by seeking experiences of "elation" that uplift the whole psyche, washing away all its frustrations, as if in one clean sweep. Rado considered this analysis not only less vague, but less condemnatory of addicted subjects—the issue is an "artificial technique" of self-regulation, not an exhaustive constitutional abnormality—and yet we can see that his analysis, like Kolb's, finds in addiction a special and indeed abnormal source of relief, which identifies the addiction as something different from the ordinary enjoyment of objects.[19]

Or consider another "classic theory" of addiction, namely, that of the sociologist Alfred Lindesmith.[20] In the late 1930s and early 1940s, Lindesmith explicitly denounced both Kolb and Rado as representatives of "the most widely accepted theory of drug addiction today," decrying their methodological lapses and the "moralistic taint" of the notion "that people become addicts, because they are inferior or abnormal and because the drug offers them an artificial support or a means of escape."[21] Yet even as Lindesmith offered a major alternative to psychological theories of addiction, he preserved their characterization of addictive attachments as unique. Lindesmith argued that addiction is what results when ordinary drug use is reinforced by "certain collective symbols" and thus, as it were, transmuted. A drug user becomes an addict only when they enter into "the culture of drug addiction," which imposes a special meaning onto drug use. No longer a simple source of pleasure, the drug is interpreted as an instrument of "magical relief," with which one can effectively control one's own affective condition. Addiction results, then, when the drug user internalizes the "symbols" that the group of addicts places upon drug-using conduct, and it is the symbolic transmutation of pleasure into magical self-determination that renders drug use irresistible, and compulsive.[22] Here we have a theory that is deeply different from Kolb's and Rado's in its content and practical implications, and yet stands alongside them as an influential site of addiction research in which the distinctiveness of addictive attachments is promoted.

As late as the 1970s, the idea that addiction is a unique form of attachment remained in the mainstream of scientific research. Consider that in 1977, for instance, NIDA research director William Pollin could introduce a volume of the agency's Research

Monograph Series devoted to psychodynamic theory by insisting that only research "focused on the structure and dynamics of total personality" could explain "why among people similarly at risk to a given drug, some will and some won't become drug dependent," and that such work thus formed a "central concern" in the field.[23] In his preface to the same volume, Heinz Kohut provided a precise explanation: like narcissists, perverts, and delinquents, the addict "suffers from a central weakness . . . in the core of his personality" and "craves the drug because the drug seems to be capable of curing the central defect in his self."[24] That "psychological disturbance" occasions the compulsive attachments of addicts was, according to the overview chapter, the "collective dictum" of the contributors, half of whom wrote again for a later volume in the series, published in 1980, which aimed "to present a representative selection of contemporary theoretical orientations and perspectives in the drug abuse research field."[25] To be sure, these volumes do not stand in for all of addiction research in the 1970s; yet they indicate that analyses of addiction as secured by a special variety of pleasure or relief were then very much still part of the scientific mainstream.

We can now specify the crucial recent shift in addiction science, which constitutes the first historical process involving a normalization of addiction. It is not that the whole field of addiction science has altered its univocal opinion; there is no such univocal view. Rather, what has happened is this: as behavioral and neuroscientific research have moved to the center of the addiction research field, the notion that addictive and nonaddictive attachments are different in kind has been displaced from the mainstream of addiction science. What is more, the rise of behavioral and neuroscientific research as the dominant perspectives in addiction science has rendered the opposite notion—that addiction is *homologous* with nonaddictive attachments—commonplace, prevalent, even presumptive in the field of addiction research. To see precisely how the rise of behavioral research and neuroscience has effected this shift, let us examine the recent history of addiction science presented in *Pathways of Addiction*, a report on the field commissioned by the NIDA in 1995 and written by a committee of the Institute of Medicine the following year.

The *Pathways* report marks the second half of the 1970s as the start of a new era for addiction research, and credits this turn to "remarkable achievements" in five domains of study: behavioral research, neuroscience, epidemiology, drug abuse prevention, and treatment.[26] Most important are behavioral research and neuroscience, for they are the basic sciences of addiction research, which define the object of the broader field. "The major contribution of behavioral research to the study of drug abuse has been the development of the self-administration model," a novel paradigm for research that casts addiction, not as a relation of meaning or a distinctive form of pleasurable object-use, but as a learned behavior like any other. In this model, addictive conduct is nothing more than highly frequent consumption and the environmental conditions that sustain this behavior at high frequency. The development of this model has not only transformed our picture of what addiction is, and how it can be studied, but also produced a new "understanding of the various causal factors that might be involved in drug abuse." If addictive conduct can be modeled and manipulated as strongly reinforced behavior, then its causes can be figured as conditions like reward timing, reward potency, and reward presentation or availability. Successful work on the basis of this perspective has "brought into question the traditional explanations of the etiology of drug abuse, such as psychopathology or various social deprivations," and bolstered the idea that addiction is better conceived as strong behavior, whose strength is explained by certain outside conditions, and not as a unique object-relation made possible by a special type of subjectivity.[27] The innovations of neuroscience have been more varied, but its most "significant progress" can be said to consist in its revelation of "the neural substrates of drug dependence."[28] If behavioral research has provided a paradigm for addiction, neuroscience has fleshed out the paradigm, and confirmed its external validity by discovering the biological means by which addictive behavior is reinforced and enacted.

Something more has happened here than the rise of a newly potent research paradigm in the addiction-science field. The new paradigm carries with it, into the mainstream of addiction research, a crucial implication, which is that addiction is an extension of normal attachment. A curious passage in *Pathways* makes this clear. Explaining how recent work in addiction science produces a new understanding of "vulnerability to repetitive drug use"—that is, vulnerability to developing an addiction—the authors write:

> Research in the area of etiology has focused on risk factors, under the assumption that some drug use is pathological. However, one of the messages from animal research using the self-administration model is that drugs easily serve as reinforcers and that conditions do not need to be pathological for drugs to be repeatedly self-administered by all animals. Research in the area of neurobiology is beginning to demonstrate that drug-taking behavior is controlled by brain mechanisms developed through evolution to ensure the reinforcing effects of biologically essential activities of eating, drinking, and copulation. The implication of these research findings is that, were it not for countervailing influences, drug use would be the norm, not an aberration.[29]

Notice the distance traveled in these few sentences. Earlier research, we learn, was based on the assumption that repetitive drug use is pathological, aberrant, uncommon; hence, the task was to determine the deviant factors (of psyche, soul, or culture) that produced the abnormal conduct. Whereas now, the leading modes of addiction research imply that were it not for countervailing forces, repetitive drug use would be the norm. Behavioral research has shown that any subject will repeatedly self-administer drugs, under normal conditions, as long as there are no strong preventative forces, and that this behavior is "easily" learned. Further, neuroscience has shown why this is true: because the behavior of repetitive drug use results from nothing more than the essential bodily processes that keep us eating, drinking, and engaging in sex. Repetitive drug use, that is, addiction, is thus identical in cause and mechanism with the most ordinary attachments, requiring no circumstantial or subjective pathology to arise. And were it not actively suppressed, addiction would be as common as the pursuit of sex, drink, and food.

The *Pathways* report captures in miniature a broader phenomenon, namely, a change in the character of addiction science as a field consequent to the rise of behavioral and neuroscience research as dominant approaches. Over the last forty years, addiction science has become a field in which the notion that addiction is homologous with normal attachment is a mainstream view. Thus, in contemporary addiction research "hijacking" circulates as the most common metaphor for what happens in addiction. The figure conveys that although addiction makes use of the same biological mechanisms as the pursuit of nourishment and sex, these mechanisms are oriented to improper ends—thus, hijacked—in an addiction. Yet what renders these ends (including but not limited to drug use) improper is a certain magnitude, not a distinctive pleasure or meaning. An NIDA pamphlet explains that "the difference between normal rewards and drug rewards can be likened to the difference between someone whispering into your ear and someone shouting into a microphone."[30] More precisely, a review of the relevant science argues, if drugs "impact natural brain reward systems to produce addiction," this means that "drugs act as natural rewards"; that drugs act *like* natural rewards but reward us "disproportionately" or in "unusually strong ways"; or they act as normal rewards but also "induce new brain processes, such as aversive withdrawal states," that overly strengthen normal processes.[31] These possible relations between drug rewards and natural rewards are "exhaustive but not mutually exclusive," and in any case they point to an essential (perhaps total) homology between addiction and normal attachment. In recent years, this homology has become more than an *implication* of mainstream work in addiction science, as the *Pathways* report put it. It is the basis for an entire domain of activity in the addiction-science field, which seeks to cast new light on the nature of our normal attachments—to food, sex, children, social partners—by taking addiction as their model.[32]

"Life is a series of addictions," we read in an article now considered seminal for research into behavioral addictions.[33] For most of the twentieth century, this would have been a marginal view, at best, or a careless metaphor, at worst. For what many of the leading scientists showed was that addiction is an aberration in the field of life, a distinctive form of attachment occasioned by an unusual formation of psyche, character, or culture. Today, the statement rings true, insofar as the homology between addiction and our relations to food, sex, social intercourse—the stuff of daily life—is a thesis accepted and explored in the mainstream of addiction science. To be sure, it may not win universal agreement, and yet its mainstream acceptance marks out one means for the normalization of addiction over the last forty years.

Diagnostic Protocols

At roughly the same time as, yet at a distance from, the developments in addiction science that we have seen, a reconceptualization of addiction in the leading diagnostic protocols normalized addiction in another way. The reconceptualization came in two phases. As the psychologists Peter Nathan, Mandy Conrad, and Anne Skinstad have shown in their history of addiction diagnosis in the United States, prior to World War II the procedures for diagnosing addiction were highly diverse and localized, determined mainly by the individual views and experiences of the physicians in charge at each institution.[34] A national protocol for addiction and other psychiatric disorders was constructed with the publication of the American Psychiatric Association's *Diagnostic and Statistical Manual for Mental Disorders* in 1952, and again with a second revision of the DSM in 1968. At this point, however, the DSM was not widely used, and its entries were all very brief, aiming only to depict the broad characteristics and etiology of each disorder, rather than to furnish detailed criteria that could tightly regulate diagnostic practice. Addiction was cataloged in its various guises—alcoholism, drug addictions—and explained as a *secondary* disorder. That is, it was classed as a subtype or "symptomatic" expression of a more basic personality disorder, which caused and explained the addiction.[35]

The first important change to this conceptualization came in 1980, with the newly written and expansive DSM-III, the revision that established the DSM as a standard clinical reference in the United States and beyond.[36] Addiction now constituted a distinct group of disorders: "Substance Use Disorders," which could be further specified as "Substance Abuse" or "Substance Dependence." Modeled on the Feighner Criteria and the Research Diagnostic Criteria, and influenced by E. M. Jellinek's typology for alcoholism, the category of Substance Use Disorders sought to specify a type of mental illness involving symptoms that were difficult to define objectively—the moment when an addiction has developed is not as clear as, say, the moment when hallucinations begin—but nonetheless belonged to a distinct pathology. Whether the DSM criteria got the threshold of addiction exactly right was not clear, but this did not matter, since they identified drug-use-related symptoms that "in almost all subcultures would be viewed as extremely undesirable." Thus, the symptoms gathered under Substance Use Disorder could be "conceptualized as mental disorders" and "distinguished from nonpathological substance use for recreational or medical purposes."[37] In short, DSM-III broke with its predecessor in conceiving addiction as its own illness, and in doing so stipulated a clear threshold between addictive and "nonpathological" substance use. A patient could be said to have crossed over into the region of illness if their pathological use constituted a "pattern"; if there was "impairment in social or occupational functioning due to substance use"; if there was a "minimal duration of disturbance of at least one month"; if there was "tolerance" or "withdrawal."[38]

The second phase of the reconceptualization, and the more important for our purposes, came with the revision of the addiction category again in the mid-1980s, which was published in 1987 in DSM-III-R. Almost immediately after the publication of DSM-III, the APA convened a Work Group to Revise DSM-III. In 1986, the members of the subcommittee tasked with revising the Substance Use Disorders category presented their proposed changes and a rationale.[39] They called for total overhaul: to collapse the distinction between Abuse and Dependence, to rewrite all existing criteria, to change the name of the category, and crucially, to replace a diagnosis that indexes a strict list of symptoms with one capable of designating a more flexible and volatile set of phenomena. These changes were needed, they argued, to correct DSM-III's inability to identify cases of addiction that involved no clear social impairment or physical withdrawal and that were mild and irregular rather than high and stable in intensity. Further, they proposed new diagnostic criteria—adopted in DSM-III-R, although without collapsing the Abuse-Dependence distinction, which would be achieved in a later edition—derived from the "dependence syndrome" model of addiction that had recently been developed as a basis for the second most influential diagnostic manual for US clinical practice, the World Health Organization's *International Classification of Diseases* (ICD).[40]

It was this adoption of the dependence syndrome model, which remains the foundation of both the DSM and ICD addiction criteria to this day, that rendered diagnostic practice one further venue for the normalization of addiction in the late 1980s. This model was first introduced in a 1976 article by the psychologists Griffith Edwards and Milton Gross.[41] Intended as an advance on existing models generally and Jellinek's approach in particular, the crucial innovations of the dependence syndrome model were two. First, against the prevailing view that addiction must be diagnosed as an "all-or-none" disease, Edwards and Gross argued that the clinical appearance of addiction is better conceived as a "syndrome," in the literal sense. Addiction is not, they argued, a distinct and stable disease entity, but rather "no more than the concurrence of phenomena," in which "not all elements need always be present, nor always with the same intensity," and about which "no assumptions need be made about the cause of the pathological process."[42] The point is not that addiction is wholly random and infinitely variable, but that its clinical appearances vary widely in etiology and presentation, and that, in general, it can only be described as a loose array of symptoms that sometimes appear together and that may wax, wane, or vanish over time. Second, in calling addiction a *dependence* syndrome, Edwards and Gross distinguished sharply between two axes of addiction too often confused: dependence, on the one hand, and disability or dysfunction, on the other. It is well known, they pointed out, that terrible consequences such as liver cirrhosis can result from drinking in the absence of dependence, while a heavily dependent person may never suffer clear physical or social impairment. Thus, they insisted that the axes be strictly separated, and that addiction diagnosis be focused on dependence, while acknowledging that dysfunction also warranted close clinical attention and treatment.

Crucial here, for our purposes, is what this model of addiction means for the distinction between addiction and nonpathological substance use. We saw that in the first two editions of the DSM, that distinction was based on a more fundamental and deeply rooted difference, between those who have and those who do not have an underlying personality disorder. And we saw that the DSM-III criteria were immediately criticized for stipulating too hard and distinct a threshold between normal use and addiction (presence of impairment, duration of one month or longer, the symptoms of tolerance and withdrawal, the consolidation of drug use into a regular pattern). The dependence syndrome, by contrast, and the criteria derived from it for ICD-9 and DSM-III-R, see the line between addiction and nonpathological substance use as blurred. Edwards and Gross make this point explicitly. After all, if addiction is "subtle and plastic rather than . . . something set hard," and if its presence must be described "in terms of degrees rather than absolutes," how can one distinguish addiction sharply from other forms of substance use, as if addiction were a single coherent state? Here is how Edwards and Gross raise the question in 1976: "In the definition of any syndrome one question must be whether the cutting point is sharp or blurred—whether the syndrome segments a continuous distribution or whether it represents an abrupt change in distribution. . . . This type of question will be answered only by further research."[43]

Edwards returned to this question over the years, and became increasingly convinced that there is no sharp cutting point. In 1981, he found that "on the basis of current knowledge, no sharp cut-off point can be identified for distinguishing drug dependence from non-dependent but recurrent drug use," and further that "there is no conceptually satisfactory cut-off point to differentiate persons exhibiting drug-related, but not syndrome-related, disabilities from the remainder of the population."[44] That is, on neither axis of addiction (dependence or disability) could such a sharp cutting point be found. Two decades later, his view remained unchanged; thus, he wrote, once the dependence syndrome model is accepted as a diagnostic paradigm, "the proper question becomes not 'Is he or she addicted to drug X?' but 'How far along the path of dependence on drug X has this person progressed?'"[45] In fact, even the metaphor of a linear progression, although better than a dichotomy of addiction and non-addiction, fails to fully capture the implication of the dependence syndrome model, since dependence is not a stable thing of which there can only be more or less, but a rough constellation which changes elements, intensity, and shape all the time.

Of course, the adoption of the dependence syndrome model as the basis for DSM-III-R and ICD-9 (and their subsequent revisions) has not entailed an *erasure* of the distinction between addicted and nonaddicted persons. After all, they are diagnostic manuals. As Edwards observes, although the model "was embraced rapidly" by them, "for classificatory purposes both DSM and ICD opted for a categorical rather than a dimensional view of dependence, and as a result lost a degree of clinical sensitivity."[46] And yet the dimensional view of the syndrome model is crucially reflected in DSM-III-R, which prefaces its list of symptoms with the warning that "It should be noted that not all nine symptoms must be present for the diagnosis of Dependence, and for some classes of psychoactive substances, certain of these symptoms do not apply," and which allows the diagnosis to be closely specified as "Mild," "Moderate," "Severe," "In Partial Remission," or "In Full Remission" according to the number and course of observed symptoms.[47] Thus, even as a line between pathology and health remains, addiction has been reconceptualized in the leading diagnostic protocols as something that *shades into* normal use, that blends in with ordinary life, and the addiction diagnosis no longer distinguishes between two essentially different kinds. This reconceptualization may thus be read as a normalization of addiction within the diagnostic field, another construction and recognition of the proximity, or better, the resemblance, between what happens in an addiction and what happens in normal experience.

Judicial Practice

That arrests for drug-related crimes continued to increase throughout the end of the twentieth century must not obscure a significant innovation that took place in US criminal justice during that same time: the construction of a new judicial outlook on the relation between drug use and criminality. According to the political scientist Ethan Nadelmann, by the mid-1980s the drug-crime connection was conceived as a cord of five strands. Heavy drug use was thought to *involve* crimes, such as possession; it was thought to *incentivize* crime, as in cases of theft intended to finance drug use; it was thought to *incite* crime, through its psychoactive effects; it was thought to *sustain* criminal organizations, such as drug cartels; and, for all these reasons, it was thought to *index* a strong tendency toward criminal acts in the heart of the heavy drug user.[48] This dense set of connections (if never made so explicit) was reflected in the figure of "the drug criminal" who appeared in political discourse especially in the 1970s and 1980s, and who appeared not just as an ordinary lawbreaker but as an "ingenious conspirator" plotting daily to "open a new door to death," someone "pilfering human dignity and pandering despair," and someone for whom "no sanctuary" could be spared in civilization—in short, as a paradigm of criminality.[49] If the notion that heavy drug use indexes deep criminality became hysterical in the words of elected officials, it was established more soberly by scholars as in this report of the National Research Council in 1987: "The empirical evidence is unequivocal that there is a link between predatory crime and drug abuse. Drug use acts as an accelerator of criminal behavior . . . [and] drug abuse is a primary indicator of the high rate offender."[50] Heavy drug use as *cause* and *sign* of criminal subjectivity.

This imagination of the heavy drug user served to justify the ramping up of policies to arrest and severely punish all instances of drug-related crime throughout the final third of the twentieth century. If even minor drug crimes were harshly punished, and the offenders confined, then the deep criminality that drug use indexed could be swept off the streets. Yet precisely this ramping up of drug-related arrests would soon lead to a rethinking of the relation between drug use and crime in the courts, which had to process and sentence the offenders arrested by the police. For as the criminologist John Goldkamp, among others, has charted, the dramatic rise in drug-related arrests in the 1980s created a practical nightmare for local courts, which were not granted the funding and staff increases enjoyed by police during the War on Drugs. The rise in arrests immediately "exacerbated already difficult problems of correctional overcrowding and court backlogs, sparking public safety concerns about drug-crime violence and raising questions among the public about the effectiveness of the justice system."[51] Facing both daily dysfunction and waning legitimacy, court officials began to see "that punitive approaches to substance abuse problems both (a) could not be indefinitely sustained by increasing imprisonment and (b) did not appear to deliver expected results in reducing drug abuse and related crime."[52] Thus, in the late 1980s, judges throughout the country became involved in experiments intended to develop a new way of conceiving and dealing with drug use in the criminal justice system.

Most consequential were the efforts of a task force led by Judge Herbert Klein in Dade County, Florida, which produced the blueprint for what is now considered by elected leaders of all stripes to be *the* most progressive and "smart" approach to addiction for criminal justice. This is the approach of "court-supervised treatment," and its institutional setting, the "drug-treatment court." To see how the development (and later dissemination) of this practice produced a novel conception of the relation between heavy drug use and crime, let us consider the classic account of the early development of court-supervised treatment authored by the drug-court judges Peggy Hora and William Schma with the attorney John Rosenthal in 1999.

According to Hora, Schma, and Rosenthal, the invention of court-supervised treatment differed from the other judicial experiments meant to relieve the burdens of drug-related cases in the late 1980s in two crucial respects. First, it differed in *aim*. Whereas most judges had simply sought better ways of processing drug-related cases, Klein and the early drug-court judges set out to solve them. That is, "instead of working on the symptoms of the increase in drug offenses (i.e., crowding of local court dockets), these courts looked for some method of curing the underlying problems of drug crimes." Hence, the invention of court-supervised *treatment* as an alternative to the "standard means of punishment and probation or parole." This would be a method, not quite for punishing crime—the traditional aim of criminal judgment—but for "correcting the addictive behavior of the drug offenders who enter the courts"—that is, for eliminating addiction.[53] Second and related, the innovators of court-supervised treatment differed in *theoretical outlook*. They set out to "view drug offenders through a different lens than the standard court system," which saw these offenders as criminals first and which construed their drug use as an expression of criminal tendencies.[54] But what if the criminality and the drug use were both signs of something deeper?

Court-supervised treatment is based on a "therapeutic" perspective that seeks to root out "the biopsychosocial cause of repeated drug use and addiction," and thereby the crimes that follow from these.[55] Although this cause was never explicitly theorized by the early drug-court leaders, it was practically constructed as a history of personal and social deprivation that has led to an under-nourishing "lifestyle" in the present. The sociologist John Nolan has argued, in an ethnographic study of drug courts, that "lifestyle," although somewhat vague, is the closest thing to a conceptualization of addiction's cause that one finds in drug-court practice; it is mentioned in the mission statements of most US drug courts, and other ethnographers have confirmed its importance as an orienting term in daily drug-court practice.[56] Roughly, it refers to a daily order and environment characterized by a lack of meaningful engagements; an abundance of unhealthy temptations; and more concretely, few chances for education, work, and family formation. Thus, court-supervised treatment figures addiction, as well as drug-related crime, as symptoms of a life mismanaged and disorganized, and not as the sign of a deep pathology or criminogenic tendency. This is why the original blueprint for court-supervised treatment—"the Miami model"—devotes just two weeks of treatment to the "preliminary goals" of "stopping drug use and ending physical dependence on the drug," and then eleven to twenty months to building "a new type of lifestyle" for the offender, as Hora, Schma, and Rosenthal put it, through individual and group counseling, GED classes, job and parenting training, and supervised placement in work settings.[57]

Since the invention of the drug court in the late 1980s, over four thousand drug courts have been created throughout the United States, and we can expect that more will arrive, given the amplified calls for their expansion with the rise of the opioid crisis.[58] Moreover, over the last few decades, court-supervised treatment has become the primary paradigm for smart criminal justice reform among elected officials across the ideological spectrum and at every level of government, and is advocated by most of the federal agencies closely involved in drug policy.[59] This does not mean, of course, that the invention and spread of court-supervised treatment has occasioned the decline of punitive responses to addiction—after all, being remanded to a drug court may be less violent as a punishment for crime than a prison sentence, but it is still punishment for crime. Nor did the invention of the drug-court model lead to an immediate and effective decrease in arrests for drug crimes; however many offenders the drug courts may have cured, the rate of arrests continued to increase at a national level for at least two decades after Klein began his work in Miami. And yet to the extent that court-supervised treatment has spread over the last thirty years, it has advanced a novel view of addiction and its relation to crime in the domain of US criminal justice. In this view, heavy drug use does not index a criminal tendency in the subject; indeed it does not index something *in* the subject at all. Rather, it reveals the presence of an ordinary person plunged into deviant conduct by a lifestyle in disrepair, and a chance for their recovery through rearrangement of daily life. Such is surely not the only view of addiction now active in US criminal justice, but it is an increasingly influential one, in wide use as a lens for drug-related crime.

At most, we can say this: the spread of court-supervised treatment and its identification as a "smart" lens for criminal justice has made it more difficult today, than it was forty years ago, to say that a criminal's drug use signals a greater danger, and thus a need for harsher punishment, than what is strictly indicated by their offense. Think here of the argument of Alfred Blumstein, who has been called "the age of Reagan's most influential criminologist."[60] Writing for *Science* in 1987, Blumstein reprised his finding, made famous a few years earlier, that "during periods of heavy drug use offenders commit crimes at frequencies six times as high as nonusing offenders," and that although the precise causal relation could not be determined, it was clear that there is a "strong association between drug use and λ [frequency of offending] for nondrug offenses." Thus although he cautioned against relying on these findings "to argue for stricter enforcement against all drug offenses"—since strict enforcement does nothing to prevent crime among "drug users who engage primarily in drug offenses"—he argued that heavy drug use "should be viewed as an aggravating factor that would warrant a more certain sentence" for "those who engage in more threatening predatory crimes like robbery and burglary."[61] Today, a history of substance use is more likely to mitigate the offense and sanction, insofar as it enables the possibility of diversion to drug court or a probation sentence based on mandatory treatment.[62] Again, the point is not that punishment has finally and completely given way to treatment. It is that the invention and spread of court-supervised treatment represents a clear, albeit not unchallenged, trend within the rhetoric and institutions of contemporary criminal justice: an increasing perception of addiction, not as an index of deep villainy, but as the sign of someone who is at bottom like anyone else, but fallen on hard times and mired in tough surroundings. Such a trend does not alone determine how addicts are identified and handled throughout the US criminal justice system, and yet it does trace, within that domain, another instance of the normalization of addiction, another linking of addiction to normal life in our time.

Policy Rhetoric

Our last process to consider is a more familiar story: the reframing of drug and addiction crises in US public-policy rhetoric over the last thirty years. Throughout the mid- and late-twentieth century, public officials routinely cast drug use and addiction not just as bodily devastations, but as ruinous of citizen virtue and thus a threat to the nation. More than despicable, drug users and addicts were conceived as degraded at the level of psyche and soul, and thus unable to carry out the preservation of family, the performance of work, and the reproduction of American values so essential for the survival of civilization. As Richard Nixon explained, to be "hooked on drugs" is to "be physically, mentally, and morally destroyed," and to replace the citizen mindset with a "drug psychology," a selfish, hedonistic psychology that is "terribly destructive of the character of [our] nation."[63] It was in this same sense that Ronald Reagan and George H. W. Bush cast drugs as "killing America," "threatening our values," and "sapping our strength as a nation."[64] In the words of drug czar William Bennett, "Using drugs is wrong not simply because drugs create medical problems; it is wrong because drugs destroy one's moral sense."[65] Thus, the *National Drug Control Strategy*, first issued under Bennett in 1989, saw a rise in addiction as "a crisis of national character," a threat to the possibility of "purposeful, self-governing society."[66] All this, and not simply hatred of the addict, justified the War on Drugs, which was a "national crusade," for President Reagan, a "just cause," for President Bush.

Clearly, this is not how the addiction crisis is conceived in national policy rhetoric today. It is not simply that medical science is now better heeded, but that the political significance of the drug problem is now cast differently: no longer a corruption of national spirit, it is strictly a deterioration of public health. Above all, it is in actual loss of life (and the societal costs of such loss) that the devastations of drug use and addiction now consist. Thus, the 2019 *National Drug Control Strategy* explains that for drug policy "the single and most important criterion of success is saving American lives" (in the literal sense) whereas thirty years ago it was reform of conduct, that is, curtailment of the *act* of drug use among the citizenry.[67] Like the epidemics of diabetes and heart disease to which it is now often analogized, an addiction crisis is a terrible tragedy, an upsurge of preventable morbidity and mortality, but not a threat to civilization.[68] The political task it occasions is not a reinforcement of citizen virtue, but the containment, at endemic levels, of a recurrent bodily disease. One can see how this rhetorical shift constitutes a further case of the normalization of addiction. Far from easily accepted, addiction is nonetheless now cast in public policy as a rate to be managed at low levels, and thus as a predictable and recurrent presence in society, one that is periodically inflamed by environmental contingencies (supply floods, loose prescription monitoring) but also finally rooted, like its sister diseases, in irreparable biological vulnerabilities.

But if the core sense and implication of this shift are clear, its timing has been obscured in recent public discourse. This must be corrected if we are to recognize the shift as a substantial transformation and not a superficial reaction to the most recent crisis. It is often said that the shift occurred during the Obama years. In fact, Obama said this himself in 2016, describing the move toward "thinking about [drug abuse] as a public health problem, and not just a criminal justice problem" as "a shift that began very early on in my administration."[69] In his familiar account, what allowed this shift to happen was the eruption of an opioid crisis whose sympathetic (white, middle- and working-class) victims made the health framing both urgent and imaginable. In the past, he explained, users and addicts were "stereotypically identified as poor, [or] minority, and as a consequence, the thinking was [drug abuse] is often a character flaw" to be punished rather than healed. But "one of the things that's changed in this opioid debate is a recognition that this [the problem of drug abuse] reaches everybody," and this has made it possible for all to see the drug problem for the health crisis that it most obviously is.

This account is not entirely wrong, but it elides a great deal. It was only with Obama and the opioid crisis that the new rhetoric was elaborated in detail and fully implemented in policy. But the shift began much earlier, in the early 1990s. By 1993, for instance, when news broke that Clinton would nominate the former police commissioner Lee Brown to become drug czar, the *New York Times* read this choice in the context of "a time when many experts are calling the heavy reliance on law enforcement of Presidents George Bush and Ronald Reagan a failure, and are pushing for big increases in spending on rehabilitation and anti-drug education." Although many hailed Brown's sensitivity to this context, the *Times* reported, "some drug experts said they were concerned that a police official might favor law-enforcement solutions to the drug problem rather than emphasize treatment and education, as many officials have been saying is needed."[70]

These concerns were reflected and assuaged in the *Interim Drug Control Strategy* issued by Brown later that year, which announced the administration's aim "to give a new sense of direction and to reinvigorate this nation's efforts against drug trafficking and abuse."[71] Essential to this new direction would be "acknowledging drug abuse as a public health problem," investing in "research to assist treatment providers to more effectively treat drug addicts," and a "move beyond ideological debates" toward "designing our anti-drug strategies based on knowledge gained from research." Also important would be to move the focus of drug policy away from disciplining "the casual and intermittent user"—fixed there by the Bush administration—onto *addicted* users, or, as they were then called, "hard-core drug users, both inside and outside of the criminal justice system, for treatment to reduce their drug use and its consequences."[72] A few years later, with Brown's replacement by Barry McCaffrey, the term "War on Drugs" would be expunged from policy discourse. As the 1997 *Strategy* explained, "the metaphor of a 'war on drugs' is misleading," both because "addressing drug abuse is a continuous challenge," whereas "wars are expected to end," and because "the United States does not wage war on its citizens, many of whom are the victims of drug abuse" and "must be helped, not defeated."[73]

This was the trend that Alan Leshner encountered and furthered when he entered the drug policy field as NIDA director in 1994. From that post, Leshner would popularize or coin many major phrases of the new political rhetoric. It was Leshner, for instance, who delivered to scholarly and popular audiences the figure of a hijacked brain in addiction, which served at once to delineate the condition of addicts and yet to render it incidental—something that might happen to anyone, and not what a few might be. It was also Leshner who made famous the phrase that he took for the title of his landmark 1997 article, "Addiction Is a Brain Disease, and It Matters," in part as a fundraising strategy whose success he had observed in his former role as acting director of the National Institute of Mental Health.[74] Equally influential was Leshner's repeated demand that "science replace ideology as the foundation of the nation's drug abuse prevention, treatment, and policy strategies."[75] Years later, "based on science, not ideology" would become the banner of the Obama administration's "21st century approach to drug policy."[76]

By the late 1990s, this new rhetoric was being broadcast on the same television networks that had helped to forge the classic images and stereotypes of the War on Drugs less than a decade earlier. As media scholars have shown, the narratives of a "siege" on middle-class, suburban neighborhoods by the drugs and drug criminals of seedy urban ghettos were built by the nightly raid footage and fearful sermons presented by trusted newscasters, as well as by the investigative reporters who claimed to have seen and confirmed the monstrous dangers of crack.[77] Thus much had changed by 1998, when viewers could listen to politicians, law enforcement officials, and university researchers advocate for a public health approach to drug policy on an episode of ABC *Nightline* entitled "It's Not a War against Drugs—It's a War against Disease." That same year, many would first encounter the new policy rhetoric in the five-part PBS documentary *Bill Moyers on Addiction: Close to Home*, which featured Leshner, McCaffrey, and many others in episodes such as "The Hijacked Brain" and "The Politics of Addiction." As one reviewer put it, "when Bill Moyers speaks, the world listens," and "the point of the series" was this: "we need to think about addiction differently, not as a failure of character but as a disease. . . . Treatment, not ostracism or punishment, is the answer."[78]

In the next decade, the new rhetoric was blended with elements of the old in federal policy, but then purified and stabilized as orthodoxy. With the election of George W. Bush and his appointment of John Walters as drug czar, some views that had been recently eliminated from the Office of National Drug Control Policy (ONDCP) reappeared. The 2003 *National Drug Control Strategy*, for instance, understood the "public health model" for drug policy to be based *both* on the "clear fact" that addiction is "a devastating disease of the brain" requiring treatment and on the earlier view that casual users, rather than addicts, are the most contagious "carriers" of spreading drug use.[79] It also took cautious distance from a trend it observed in European countries to "frame the drug issue as a public health rather than a law enforcement problem," preferring to mix the two approaches.[80] But by 2006, the *Strategy* would drop this latter point, and the concern with casual users would also soon disappear. In 2009 the Bush administration released its final version of the report, still prepared under Walters, where it fully installed the public health outlook as a "pillar of the *National Drug Control Strategy*," encompassing "two principles: 1) addiction is a disease, and 2) addiction is treatable."[81]

The consolidation of the new rhetoric by the late 2000s, but
before the Obama years, is also reflected in the "evolution" of public officials. When Walters was appointed in 2001, many decried
the return to office of the man who had been William Bennett's
second-in-command throughout the War on Drugs. As one critic
put it, "John Walters stands for the proposition that drug policy
has nothing to do with science or public health. It's all about punishment."[82] Yet even as marijuana arrests did peak during Walters's time, by 2008 he would open his response to public questions about drug policy by noting that "I think it is important
that we put this in context: addiction is a public health issue that
affects millions of Americans who either suffer with the disease,
have a loved one who is addicted, are the victims of crimes per-
petrated by addicted individuals."[83] One year prior and across the
aisle, then-senator Joe Biden, who in 1993 had organized a Judiciary Committee report castigating the Bush administration for
under-funding police and military operations in the War on Drugs,
introduced a bill that would have written the new rhetoric into
law: the Recognizing Addiction as a Disease Act of 2007.

What, then, of the influence of the opioid crisis? By the end of
Bush's tenure, it was clear that prescription drug abuse had become
something more than what in 2005 was only "an emerging drug
abuse problem."[84] And just two years after Bush's departure from
office, the Centers for Disease Control and Prevention (CDC) would
declare that prescription painkiller overdoses in this country had
reached epidemic levels. Since then, the shocking numbers of the
opioid crisis have not just amplified but reinforced the changes in
drug policy rhetoric that began in the 1990s, having made more urgent the need for a political framing that might help to avert further
loss of life. But they were not among the numbers named by President Bush in his final radio address on drug policy, which he ended
with the story of a former addict, now a professional athlete, who

> shows that the devastation of drug addiction can happen to
> anyone—but that with faith and determination, anyone can
> turn a life around. So today I ask every American with a drug or
> alcohol problem to seek treatment—because your life is precious
> to the people who love you, our Nation needs your contribu-

tions, and there is a more hopeful future ahead. I ask all Americans to reach out to your neighbors in need—and do your part to help our Nation win the fight against illegal drugs.[85]

Surely the opioid crisis has had an effect on how we speak, but it did not invent the rhetorical conventions that Bush draws upon here. These conventions emerged thirty years ago, when the drug problem was reimagined not only as a matter of disease, but in the terms of public health: as involving a form of suffering that, as Bush puts it, can happen to anyone; as amenable to relief through prevention and treatment, rather than requiring a restoration of national spirit; and as a hazard to be held at a baseline, not a fire to be extinguished. No longer a pestilence, the spread of addiction is now conceived as being more like an economic slump or natural disaster, as Obama has put it: a terrible emergency, yet a recurrent possibility, a devastation that we lament yet can expect to find again in the kind of life that is ours.[86]

We thus find normalization at work in four of the most important developments of American knowledge about addiction over the last forty years. The narrative form of normalization does not exhaust these developments, but it does fit and comprehend them, and what is more, it reveals their shared significance. For all their differences, the mainstreaming of behavioral and neuroscientific paradigms in addiction science, the incorporation of the dependence syndrome model in leading diagnostic manuals, the dissemination of court-supervised treatment in criminal justice, and the recasting of addiction crises as problems of public health in national political rhetoric all construct addiction—and this in departure from the theories, idioms, and models that had earlier prevailed in each of these domains—as normal, and figure the addict as a normal subject, akin to any other human if not in the literal facts of their behavior, then in their deep character, nature, and kind. It follows that normalization is not an isolated process but a recurrent one, even an increasingly common process, in our recent history. Normalization can thus be reckoned as one crucial trend of knowledge about addiction in our time. I would like to close this chapter by reflecting on the questions raised by the existence of such a trend among us. These will be the driving questions of all the remaining chapters; hence, I lay them out in some detail.

One question is about the timing of normalization's emergence as a widespread process or trend. We have seen that the various instances of normalization occurred in a diverse range of domains and were driven by diverse local actors and motivations. And although there have been some mutual influences between them, none has fully caused any other. The neuroscience of addiction, for instance, has been incorporated into the public-health rhetoric of state policy, but it did not produce the latter.[87] Nor do the conventionally cited meta-influences on thinking about addiction in the late twentieth century—the rise of prescription opioid overdoses among whites starting at the end of the 1990s, the rising profile of biomedical knowledge of addiction in public discourse achieved through the promotional activities of the NIDA starting in the mid-1990s[88]—explain the *emergence* of normalization as a trend, since the latter preceded them. (Of course, the "whitening face" of addiction and the popular biomedicalization of addiction may well have *extended* the trend of normalization.) How, then, can we understand the fact that all four of our instances of normalization arose or were consolidated at almost the same time, that is, in the long 1980s? This need not be resolved into a causal question. Rather, we can make a more open-ended inquiry: What else was going on, in the last two decades of the twentieth century in American culture and society, that may have promoted the idea that addiction is a normal part of human experience, and that the addict is like any other human, wherever it happened to emerge? To narrow our search, I will put the question this way: What cultural and social trends concerning the depiction and understanding of human desire, self-control, and motivation in the late twentieth-century United States may have indirectly promoted the normalization of addiction?

A second question is about the effect or consequence of normalization, conceived as a trend. It is, of course, relatively easy to imagine the effects of normalization *within* each domain where it has occurred. We have already seen, for instance, how the normalization of addiction in science not only reflects but spurs the use of addiction as a paradigm for desire and attachment more generally in contemporary neuroscience research. And clearly, normalization in clinical diagnostics changes the relationship between doctor and patient, who are no longer divided by a difference of psychological kind, as well as the meaning and range of practical application for addiction diagnoses. But this chapter has shown us that normalization has occurred in a range of domains at once, in our society; and indeed, in the chapters to come we will encounter a number of further means by which addiction has become normalized over the last forty years. And this raises the question of whether there are broad cultural effects that can be attributed to the trend of normalization as a whole. What consequences follow from the fact that so many of our sources of knowledge about addiction now cast it as, or as akin to, normal experience? What new ways of seeing and describing our desire, our will, and our selfhood are promoted, when addiction is increasingly understood to be normal? What older ways are lost, or demoted?

These questions are raised by the historical overview of the normalization of addiction that this chapter has offered. They can only be deepened, however, by shifting the focus of our analysis. In this chapter, we have traced and found recurrent the basic pattern of normalization. We now need to look more closely at the results of normalization, or more precisely, at the understanding of normal life, and of the normal subject, that it yields. To do this, we will narrow our focus in subsequent chapters to single instances or aspects of normalization, and examine in detail how they figure and construct the human, and human experience, in such a way as to render them compatible with, and inclusive of, the possibility of addiction. Doing so will reveal normalization in a new light. We will no longer be reading it only as a recasting of addiction, but also as a recasting of the human subject, and of the shape and substance of human life. And seen in this light, the pattern of normalization will appear to us as a process of rethinking the human subject that, at least in its broad contours, we can find occurring elsewhere in late twentieth-century American society and culture, in domains beyond the science, medicine, and politics of addiction, including psychotherapy, digital technology, and personal health. Thus, the one shift of focus—attending, now, to the figure of the human that emerges through the normalization of addiction—will lead to a second shift: an attentiveness to the parallels between the normalization of addiction and other recent social and cultural changes affecting how desire, motivation, and selfhood are understood in American society. Examining these parallels will be my method for clarifying the timing and consequence of normalization's emergence as a trend over the last forty years.

TWO

The Power of
Behavioral Interventions

This chapter dwells on a practical instance of the normalization of addiction. This is the rise, over the last thirty years, of *behavioral interventions* (or, synonymously, *behavioral therapies*) as the leading modality of addiction treatment in American society. In characterizing behavioral interventions as *leading*, I mean to indicate, first, their commonality in our time. Today, if one seeks out addiction treatment, one is most likely to be offered some form of behavioral therapy. As federal survey data show, the vast majority of treatment facilities "frequently" utilize such behavioral interventions as cognitive behavior therapy (94%) and motivational interviewing (93%), while only around 38 percent of facilities offer medications (the main alternative to behavioral interventions) such as naltrexone and buprenorphine.[1] As the National Institute on Drug Abuse and the Office of the Surgeon General report, "Behavioral therapies . . . are the most commonly used forms of drug abuse treatment."[2] Yet behavioral interventions are not only common in our time. They are often seen as the most effective form of treatment. This statement may seem to clash with the familiar claim that medication-assisted treatment, or MAT, is the "gold standard" of addiction treatment, but let us remember that, as the Surgeon General's Report on addiction explains, "The combination of behavioral interventions and medications to treat substance use disorders is commonly referred to as MAT."[3] And in this combination, the medication serves to enable and support behavioral interventions, which are primary. The Surgeon General's Report analogizes "medications for substance use disorders" to "insulin for patients with diabetes." Both control acute symptoms—surges of craving in one case, hyperglycemia in the other—whereas behavioral therapies (addiction) and diet change (diabetes) serve as the "broader disease control strategy."[4] According to the NIDA, "Medications are an important *element* of treatment for many patients, especially when combined with counseling and other behavioral therapies."[5] In short, behavioral interventions are now what most addicts get, and what they are said to most need.

The psychiatrists Kathleen Carroll and Lisa Onken, both leading researchers in the field of drug-abuse treatment, have set down the basic historical coordinates for the rise of behavioral interventions. By the late 1980s, techniques such as cognitive behavior therapy and contingency management, initially developed outside the addiction field, were being used in many addiction treatment settings. Yet their use was uncoordinated, lacked theoretical justification, and "there was continued pessimism in the field regarding the efficacy of behavioral therapies for drug use disorders." The situation changed "in the early 1990s," when a new funding program directed by the NIDA actively promoted the use and legitimacy of behavioral therapies by supporting "behavioral treatment development, spanning from origination and initial testing of novel behavioral therapies to their dissemination in community settings."[6] Throughout the 1990s, studies of behavioral therapies— their process, mechanism, and outcomes—"began to appear more frequently in the drug abuse treatment literature," and this gave behavioral therapies a new status, which they still enjoy today: an evidence-based treatment modality.[7] All this occurred at a time when public officials, seeking distance from the policy framework of the War on Drugs, laid increasing emphasis on promoting and disseminating evidence-based treatments as a primary response to addiction. Thus, the 1990s were the crucial decade in which behavioral interventions developed in three ways: first, they were defined and theorized as having a shared therapeutic approach; second, they were legitimated by a growing outcome literature, including studies based on randomized trials; third, they became more common. All three developmental outcomes—increased integrity, legitimacy, and commonality—persist in our time; thus, the early 1990s to the present can be considered the period of behavioral interventions' rise.

This chapter reads the rise and dissemination of behavioral interventions as an instance of the normalization of addiction. As I will show, the various techniques of behavioral interventions are coordinated by a medical theory that figures the addict as subjectively normal in spite of their disease. On this theory, addiction involves normal volitional processes that have, for temporary reasons, become attached to an overly narrow range of objects. The task of treatment is thus to widen that range of objects, and this is achieved not by reforming the will of the addict, which remains normal in mechanism and quality, but by deliberately attaching the addict to more and healthier objects through methods to be seen. The rise of behavioral interventions circulates this normalizing knowledge of addiction in two ways. First, insofar as that rise encompasses not just the increasing *use* of behavioral interventions, but the growth of an academic and professional literature that articulates why and how behavioral interventions work as treatment, it disseminates the theory that underlies this treatment modality in journal articles, pamphlets, and practitioner handbooks. And second, the increasing use of behavioral interventions itself spreads the theory that underlies it as a basic knowledge for those who give and receive treatment, both because the practical use of any treatment requires describing its therapeutic premises and because the very structure and process of a treatment convey those same premises. Thus, we can consider the rise of behavioral interventions, which I will cast synoptically as the spread of a practice or method of power, as in part the spread of a normalizing knowledge of addiction, as it constructs the addict as a suffering yet normal subject in both erudite literatures and quotidian settings.

This reading of behavioral interventions as extending the normalization of addiction will be the basis for a second interpretation, which is the main task of this chapter. If the techniques of behavioral intervention figure the addict as constitutionally normal in spite of their disease, they represent techniques for reforming and transforming conduct that do not require stipulating deep individual abnormality. Conceived this way, behavioral interventions appear as something more than a new mode of addiction treatment. They appear as *post-disciplinary* methods of subject-construction and control, that is, methods that represent and reform human conduct without any of the characteristics that Foucault gathered under the rubric of discipline: projection and judgment of a deep personal character as the underlying source of all conduct; an ambition to change conduct, accordingly, through a reform of deep character; and hence use of technical procedures intended to remake character and soul. This interpretation of behavioral therapies as post-disciplinary in imagination, ambition, and method is important insofar as it reveals the rise of this new modality of addiction treatment, and its normalization of addiction, as part of a larger historical process that has attracted the interest of many social and political theorists in recent years.[8] This is the waning of discipline as a dominant modality of power in late-modern American society, a process that has been traced by others across the domains of work, political economy, and punishment, each of which has featured the rise of methods for reforming conduct without knowing or acting on individual characters since the late twentieth century. Seeing behavioral interventions as post-disciplinary methods—as methods that promise to eliminate unwanted conduct yet presume the inner normalcy of the subject that they treat—casts the domain of addiction treatment as another site where discipline loses its hold in late-modern American society and where new methods of subject-construction and control are emergent in our time. And this allows us to begin setting our instances of the normalization of addiction in a broader cultural context, and to see what trends in the imagination and governance of the subject may be revealed, as well as furthered, by the ways of constructing the addict that we are examining.

   To develop both interpretations, this chapter stages a contrast between the modality of behavioral interventions and another modality of treatment, which was popular in an earlier time: the therapeutic community (TC). To avoid misunderstanding, let me underscore here that in this chapter, the main relation between behavioral interventions and TCs is conceptual, not historical.

Of course, as the historian Claire Clark has charted, the popularity of TCs as a treatment mode in the United States began to fall just as behavioral interventions began to rise in prominence and prestige—that is, in the early 1990s.[9] Many of the reasons for this coincidence are clear, including changes in the health care landscape that increasingly privileged short-term, outpatient treatments over the long-term, residential approach of TCs, and new funding regulations instituted in the late 1980s that privileged forms of treatment compatible with training in the social work, psychology, and mental health fields.[10] Thus, it is roughly true that what the treatment expert Fernando Perfas has described as "the decline of the large traditional TCs" since the late 1980s is almost immediately followed by the rise of behavioral interventions.[11] However, although TCs were certainly one of the leading modalities of addiction treatment through the 1980s—as late as 1989, we read in a national survey of drug abuse treatment that "the three major 'modalities' or types of treatment currently being administered are the outpatient methadone clinics, therapeutic communities, and outpatient drug-free programs"[12]—they were simply that: *one* of the leading modalities. It would be inaccurate, then, to see the relation between TCs and behavioral interventions as one of strict historical succession, in which one dominant modality is displaced by another.

Fortunately, that historical perspective is not needed in this chapter. In what follows, the TC figures, not as the predecessor of behavioral interventions, but as a modality of treatment that is incompatible with the latter at the most basic, conceptual level, and which thus illuminates by way of contrast what is distinctive about behavioral intervention. As we will see, TC treatment was exactly premised on an interpretation of addictive conduct as symptomatic of an abnormal will, rooted in the under- or maldeveloped character of the addict-subject. Hence, it was a form of treatment that aimed at *reforming the personality* of individuals, or *altering the character type* that underlies addiction.[13] Further, it was a form of treatment that used techniques that facilitate knowledge of, and influence upon, deep subjective character. These included placement of each patient within a graduated social hierarchy that measured and publicized the maturity and self-possession of the patient, as well as therapy sessions designed to facilitate the internalization of new values and personality ideals. Of course, the fact that TCs were an actual, popular form of treatment just before the spread of behavioral interventions lends it special value as a contrasting treatment modality. For it means that there are, among the patients now subjected to behavioral intervention, some who would have, just forty years earlier, been subjected to TC treatment. The number of such patients measures the extent to which the relation between TCs and behavioral interventions really is one of historical succession. But the primary analytic value of the TC in this chapter lies in the fact that it realizes, in an actually existing form, a fully disciplinary mode of addiction treatment. Thus, it provides a background against which to show the precise senses in which behavioral interventions are normalizing and post-disciplinary.

I turn now to an analysis of the TC structure and technique, and follow this with a study of behavioral interventions. I then reflect on the significance of the rise of a normalizing and post-disciplinary method of treatment in our time, considering it not just as a major development for the contemporary construction of addicts, but as part of the rising of post-disciplinary power as a broad cultural condition in late-modern American society.

In examining the TC, my interest is selective. During the height of its popularity, the TC differed from the other major modalities of addiction treatment in several important respects, including its client base, its cost, its employment of ex-addict staff, and its setting within residential facilities. For our purposes, however, what was most importantly distinctive about the TC was its ambition to correct the symptoms of addiction by reforming the *subject* of addiction. As George De Leon, an early researcher of TCs who would become one of the most prominent national advocates for TC treatment, put it, the aim of such treatment is not just elimination of drug use, but a change in "the whole person" behind the conduct.[14] Or, as the founder of an early TC which would become a model for later facilities wrote, TC treatment is aimed at "reforming a human personality."[15] Or again, in the words of an ex-TC client, advocating for TC funding before the US House in 1986, what the TC provided her was a new individuality: with treatment, she insists, "it was like a new person was emerging from myself"; now, "I can finally say that Lee Ann [that is, the speaker] is an individual."[16] This orientation of the TC toward transforming the individual is what rendered it an instance of disciplinary treatment, and it is the focus of our examination of TCs.

In what follows, I draw my account of TC treatment from *Therapeutic Communities for Addictions*, a 1986 volume of essays authored by researchers and practitioners, which aimed to codify the dynamic yet distinctive "concept, model, and methods" of the TC.[17] The first volume of its kind, *Therapeutic Communities for Addictions* gathered leading advocates such as George De Leon (a coeditor of the text), Maxwell Jones, and Harry Wexler, and was, in the words of its reviewers, "long-awaited" by practitioners, "balanced and comprehensive," and, as intended by the editors, "representative of the current thinking about therapeutic communities."[18] Although the actual practices of different TC facilities surely varied, TC treatment nonetheless designated a unique and coherent approach to dealing with addiction. As the opening chapter of *Therapeutic Communities for Addictions* explains, this approach involves a distinctive *process* and *structure* of treatment.

Consider first the "process." Most often, TC treatment was organized as a sequence of three stages. First was "Induction," or assimilation into the TC facility. Second, and the longest and most intensive of the three, was "Primary Treatment." Finally came "Re-Entry," involving supervised reintegration into the wider society following Primary Treatment. Crucially, Primary Treatment was further divided into three sub-stages. All sub-stages involved a daily regimen of work duties (cooking, cleaning, and the like), group meetings, encounter therapy, counseling, and community management (this last referred to the dispensation of punishments and privileges for violations of, or compliance with, treatment requirements—discipline, in the ordinary sense). But the sub-stages were graduated, and as one moved from, say, sub-stage II to sub-stage III, the precise details of one's daily regimen would be modified to match one's treatment progress and needs. And to facilitate these intermediate graduations, the staff regularly assessed the extent to which residents had "internalized the TC's perspective and commitment to change" and shown "personal growth . . . , emotional stability, and [increases in] self-esteem."[19] If a resident showed sufficient progress in internalizing TC values and growth of personality, they would be moved to the next sub-stage of Primary Treatment, bringing better work details, more privileges, and new roles in peer counseling and group meetings. This continual but graduated movement through treatment composes a "developmental process" that facilitates "the evolution of a socially responsible, personally autonomous individual." What allows a resident to move from one stage (or sub-stage) to the next, and thus what each stage is intended to achieve, is "increased maturity and personal autonomy."[20] As should be clear, the TC process is designed to recapitulate the process that leads from infantile helplessness to adult autonomy, and treatment is isomorphic with maturation. Thus, in the TC one speaks equally of "'getting well' or 'growing up,'" and the trajectory of TC treatment "enables the individual to grow up and develop emotionally, socially, culturally, ethically, morally, sexually, and vocationally."[21] The relation between TC and childhood development is not metaphorical, but homological: TC treatment is "consistent with the normal process of growing up."[22]

Hence the "structure" of the TC as a "new family."[23] Just as childhood development can occur only within the milieu of a family, TC treatment is set in a pyramidal structure in which members ("People in a Therapeutic Community are members, as in any family setting, not patients"[24]) are subordinate to higher-stage members, who are like older siblings, and staff, who are the parents of the family. The TC is composed of "stratified communities of peer groups," in which members at higher strata serve as "role models" for those at lower levels. Meanwhile, all the communities of peer groups are under the watch and direction of the staff, the "parental surrogates," who manage the TC "as an autocracy," providing order and stability. In short, the TC's "social organization is a family surrogate system, vertically stratified," offering both the upward mobility and strict regulation needed for the development of personal maturity and individuality.[25]

Why this homology between addiction treatment and the development of children into autonomous individuals? The answer appears in one of the essays in *Therapeutic Communities for Addictions*, which aims to synthesize, into a coherent narrative, explanations of TC treatment offered in the research literature up to the mid-1980s. Although the etiology of addiction varies to some degree, and addictions to different substances tend to arise by varying means, we learn that "most residents of therapeutic communities belong to the character disorder type of heroin addicts."[26] That is, most TC residents are heroin addicts, and for the most part their addictions can be viewed as expressions of disorders at the level of character or personality. Hence, this is the etiology reflected and addressed by the design of TC treatment and that had been featured in most studies of TCs. Here is how this etiological story goes:

"Dependence on the effect of heroin . . . can be seen as an adaptation to an impaired ego-development." Addiction, then, reveals a hindrance in the actual early development of the addict, and it is an adaptation to that hindrance. In particular, addiction is an adaptation to a hindrance that occurs "in the separation/individuation stage" of development, which is "the period in which feelings of self-esteem, control of impulses, and super-ego function are developed." The cause of the hindrance "can be found in the family situation" at the time of separation/individuation. Most likely, "the child received inconsistent messages and unclear limits were set to his behavior," or "the parents were frequently absent and often there was a serious emotional deprivation." Either way, the pathological condition is *absence or inconsistent presence of parents*, which results in three forms of deprivation for the child: lack of love and affirmation; lack of limits on conduct; and lack of clear principles by which to regulate behavior. (Put technically, the result is "absence of an internalization of positive object relations and an impaired super-ego development.") With time, the child grows, but never develops the psychic resources that enable normal individuals to develop refined control over conduct: a self-worth based, and thus dependent, upon the approval of others; an inner voice that pushes one to pursue what is right, not just what is pleasurable; and a motive, in the form of guilt, to heed that inner counsel. This mal-development comes to a head at the time of "separation from the parent's home in late adolescence." Lack-

ing capacities for moral self-regulation and pursuit of higher pleasure, the grown child enters the social world with painful feelings
of self-hatred, no interest in culture, mature love, or work, and a
tendency toward "behavior [that] is aimed at immediate gratification" which was never conquered. Now, the developmental hindrance calls forth an adaptation in the form of drug abuse. "Use
of drugs can meet the need for affection, and [need for] support
from a parent can be met immediately" by the same means. The
addict is dependent on drugs because they have no other way of
seeking comfort and pleasure in adult reality, while others procure
these from internalized objects, moral self-regulation, and social
productivity.[27]

This is why TC treatment resembles childhood development.
It is another development, a do-over, that aims to eliminate addiction not through an isolated attack on addictive conduct, but
by producing a more mature individual, and thereby altering the
overall *style* of acting—the will to immediate gratification, the
lack of any will to do otherwise—that addictive conduct realizes
and reveals. Hence, TC treatment begins by placing the addict in a
closed reality where they can become a child again—surrounded by
siblings; assigned chores, daily schedules, punishments, and privileges; under the watch of autocratic yet compassionate parents—
and it ends by staging a return to social reality, a recapitulation
of late adolescence, in which the individual can finally "separate
from his new family in a healthy way."[28] Every aspect of the TC
process and structure is meant to facilitate this restaging of infancy, development, and separation from the family. The figuring
of advanced members as "role models" and staff as "parental surrogates" is meant to facilitate, through identification and intro-
jection, the psychic resources that never obtained in the addict's
first childhood, that is, to "create different identification from that
toward [original] parents," and to form "positive introjections . . .
producing an increase of self-esteem, insight, and trust."[29] The use
of work assignments, punishments and privileges, and emphasis
on household duties is meant to instill "important values . . . such
as honesty, concern, and responsibility" as a moral code in members.[30] The tripartite process of treatment is meant to repeat the
structure and not just the trajectory of childhood: Stage I, Induction, provides the addict (infant) with a feeling of "support and

security"; Stage II, Primary Treatment, gives the addict (child) a sense of "order and responsibility," a capacity to "take responsibilities," and "a growing feeling of entitlement as he experiences to be of value to someone else"; and Stage III, Re-Entry, allows the burgeoning individual (adolescent) to experiment in the real world, trying out jobs and meeting with friends and family, to "seek their own identity . . . as if they were adolescents again," in order finally to go out into the world once again, but this time with the resources to redirect and resist the childhood will toward immediate and cheap gratification.[31]

Let us step back and underscore three crucial features of TC treatment, which will be the basis for a comparison with behavioral interventions below.

(1) The TC does not conceive addiction as an isolated object-relation, but as one instance of a disturbed way of acting, an abnormal will, on the part of the addicted subject: a will to immediate comfort and gratification that is not regulated by morals, super-egoic demands, or desire for higher pleasures. Addiction reflects "a disorder of the whole person, affecting some or all areas of functioning"—a wide range of conduct, not just pursuit of drugs.[32]

(2) The TC conceives this abnormal will not as a sign of criminality or evil, but as the result of an impaired development of the addict's ego, "I," or character. The root of the addiction is an abnormal character or individuality; hence TC treatment is meant to achieve "a global change in the individual," or a production of the subject as a fully formed individual. Its ideal is a normative model of the human person.[33]

(3) The technical instruments of the TC are intended to gain access to, and operate on, the deep character and personality of members. These include the stratified, autocratic family structure; the regular examination of individual values and maturity; the use of work, punishments, and privileges to test and stimulate members' capacities for social responsibility, moral deliberation, and restraint on the will to gratification. Most broadly, the technical instruments are meant to reproduce the natural drivers of psychic growth and development: the various aspects of life in a family.

These three features clearly characterize TC treatment as both abnormalizing and disciplinary in imagination and technique. This is not to say that TC treatment simply denigrates or condemns its members, or that we ought to consider it unitarily or ultimately punitive rather than genuinely therapeutic. It is rather to say that an essential feature of TC treatment was its construction of addiction as the sign of an abnormal will (to use slightly less pejorative terms, we can say, an immature will), and its construction of an abnormal will, in turn, as part of an abnormal character, "I," or individuality. Hence, it conceived the trajectory of treatment as a movement in which the subject was made more normal, more compatible with the ideal of what an adult human person should be. Related, TC treatment was disciplinary, not just in the ordinary sense, but also in its therapeutic rationality: it comprised a set of techniques that sought to reform conduct by reforming the individual, and that acted on the core of the subject—that is, on the addict's inner character or personality.

Just four decades ago, TC treatment was still among the major modalities of addiction treatment in American society.[34] Although TCs have not disappeared since that time, they have certainly been marginalized, and in important ways "hybridized," or "fused with other treatment models" in order to survive a novel health care and addiction treatment landscape.[35] They have also lost their cultural prominence over the last thirty years. A recent book on the history of TCs observes that the invention and advocacy of TC treatment has "mostly dropped out of our drug-policy origin stories."[36] In the early 1980s, Nancy Reagan routinely cited her visit to Daytop Village, one of the early TCs, as having first sparked her interest in the issue of drug abuse.[37] As we turn to examine what has become the leading modality of addiction treatment in our time, bear in mind this disciplinary treatment that was in wide use until recently, for this will help us to apprehend the specificity and significance of what behavioral interventions have brought into being.

Let me approach behavioral interventions by an indirect route, which will help illuminate their role and importance in our world. In 2017, a case before the Massachusetts Supreme Court attracted wide attention as an apparent test of whether treatment could finally replace punishment for those caught in the grip of the criminal justice system. As the *Atlantic* reported, "support for increased access to treatment and reduced reliance on incarceration" for addicts "is not, in the main, controversial in 2017—not politically and not medically," but it had not yet "translated to the courts." *Commonwealth v. Eldred* was an "illustration of this disconnect" as well as a chance to make the translation.[38] The editorial board of the *New York Times* agreed, seeing in *Eldred* a "potential to usher in a welcome change to drug control policies across the country" and a test of the legal basis for "policies that punish relapse with jail time and keep sufferers from proven treatments."[39] Speaking to *NPR*, the chief legal counsel for the Massachusetts Bar Association predicted that the case would move state lawmakers to increase funding for addiction treatment, as it would eliminate jails, moving forward, as a ready destination for offenders diagnosed with addiction.[40] In short, *Commonwealth v. Eldred* was widely viewed as making the legal case for replacing punishment, even in the criminal justice system, with evidence-based treatments as the primary social response to addiction.

My interest here is not in the outcome of *Eldred*, which realized none of the promise that commentators had anticipated, both because the Massachusetts Supreme Court ruled against the defendant and because in doing so the Court qualified its ruling in such a way as to avoid taking a stand on whether punishment is an appropriate response to addiction. Rather, my interest is in the argument of the defendant's brief, and in the science that the brief relies on. Together, they show us, first, that behavioral interventions are now conceived not just as a leading mode of therapy for addiction, but as a "best practice," as the brief puts it, for transforming the conduct of addicts; and second, how behavioral interventions reshape conduct without reliance on punitive means.[41]

To grasp this argument, we need a bit of the case history. In mid-2016, Julie Eldred was arrested and arraigned on a charge of larceny. Eldred admitted guilt and explained that she had stolen jewelry in order to buy heroin, to which she was addicted. In exchange for her admission of guilt, the judge issued a "continuance without a finding." This allowed Eldred to serve a one-year probation term, which, if fulfilled successfully, would lead to a dismissal of the case. Since Eldred had cited heroin use as the motive for her crime, the judge "required her to remain drug free, submit to random drug screens, and attend outpatient substance abuse treatment three times each week."[42] Eldred entered treatment, but soon after failed a drug test administered by her probation officer. The judge decided that Eldred would need to enter inpatient treatment in order to continue with probation. While Eldred's attorney sought an open bed at an inpatient facility, Eldred would be held in jail. The search took ten days, and Eldred was jailed for that time, before being moved to the treatment facility.

It is this jail sentence that Eldred and her attorney were challenging as cruel and unusual, and hence illegal.[43] The basis for this argument was their assertion that punishment is "clinically contraindicated" in two senses.[44] First, punishment *obstructs* treatment. Although some prisons and jails do offer in-house treatment services, for the most part being incarcerated means that one is in a setting inconducive to healing one's addiction. Second, punishment *worsens* addiction. It is, after all, well known that addictive cravings are heightened by experiences of stress, anxiety, and isolation, all of which are inevitable results of incarceration. But the fact that punishment is not healing is not enough to make it so cruel as to be illegal. Thus, the defendant's brief adds a further point, which is that in the last thirty years, advances in addiction treatment have yielded therapeutic techniques that not only heal the addict, but also control the conduct of addicts much more effectively than existing methods of punishment. And *this* is what renders punishment indefensible, since it is no longer just an obstacle to healing, but also an ineffective method for conduct reform compared with new addiction treatments. Given the "significant advances in 'evidence-based' treatment approaches" over recent decades, the use of punishment in response to addiction no longer has any justification.[45] In the words of the brief, "in the light of our contemporary understanding of substance use disorder as a chronic, relapsing, and *eminently treatable* brain disease, mandating that Eldred remain drug free and then jailing her when she 'fails to comply' is cruel, arbitrary, and fundamentally unfair."[46] No longer our most effective means of controlling unwanted conduct, punishing an addict now lacks any basis but cruelty.

It is here that *Eldred* casts behavioral interventions as a leading mode of social response to addiction. To show that punishment is not just harsh but ineffective, the brief offers a direct comparison between "the inefficacy of punishment" and "the efficacy of current evidence-based approaches to drug addiction treatment." We learn that these approaches are two:

> On the psychotherapeutic level, effective treatments include motivational interviewing, cognitive behavioral therapy, and contingency management, each of which is "positive-oriented and non-judgmental." On the pharmacological level, opioid agonists such as buprenorphine have been shown to be effective in "helping patients achieve disease remission," "in some ways like insulin for patients with diabetes." "Whether treating diabetes or substance use disorder," however, medication is most effective when used "as part of a broader treatment plan involving behavioral health therapies and recovery support services."[47]

In other words, the two approaches are *behavioral interventions* (in the sources cited for this passage, all the examples of psychotherapeutic treatments given in the main text are explicitly named as "behavioral interventions") and *medications*. But the two are not equal, since, as the brief rushes to add, medications are effective as *part* of broader treatment plans that make use of behavioral therapies.[48] Thus, it is behavioral interventions that promise to obviate, indeed render obsolete, not only older methods of treatment, but also punishment. It is behavioral interventions that would have been promoted if, as the news coverage of *Eldred* had anticipated, this case had become the occasion for advancing the replacement, in our society, of punishment for addicts by evidence-based treatments.

Having illustrated their promise and status, let us examine more closely how behavioral interventions work, and what distinguishes them as a mode of treatment. To do this, I want to turn now to one of the sources, or "authorities," referenced many times in the brief. The evidentiary value of this source is twofold. First, of all the texts that the brief cites for its claims about contemporary treatment, this is the source that offers the most thorough explanation of the logic and practice of behavioral interventions. Second, this source is an article coauthored by the director of the NIDA, the director of the National Institute on Alcohol Abuse and Alcoholism, and the former deputy director of the Office of National Drug Control Policy and published in the *New England Journal of Medicine*. Hence, although it does not discuss how behavioral treatment might vary in actual practice, we can take it as a reliable statement of how behavioral interventions are conceptualized by some of the leading authorities on addiction treatment in our time.

Although the title of the article, "Neurobiologic Advances in the Brain Disease Model of Addiction," has the ring of a straightforward scientific review article, this piece is in fact closely tailored to the argument that we have been following in Eldred's brief. That is, it reviews recent advances in addiction science and treatment in order to make the case that punishment ought to be abandoned as a first-line social response to addiction. It opens with the claim that "centuries of efforts to reduce addiction and its related costs by punishing addictive behaviors [have] failed to produce adequate results." A key goal of the article is to advocate "more effective methods of prevention and treatment," namely, behavioral interventions.[49] Thus, the science it reviews is not any and all research on addiction, brain, and behavior, but rather specific findings that can help correct the views of those who oppose abandoning punishment as a response to the conduct of addicts. These opponents tend to fear that to replace punishment with treatment is effectively to license socially unwanted conduct, "excusing personal responsibility and criminal acts instead of punishing harmful and often illegal behaviors." Conventional ideas "about self-determination and personal responsibility" cast unwanted conduct as the result of individual decisions that are not sufficiently sensitive to the consequences of such conduct. These ideas lead some to believe that punishment, or the application of painful or negative consequences for conduct, is the best and most appropriate way of eliminating antisocial behaviors.[50] But these ideas are mistaken. In fact, the authors advocate the use of evidence-based treatments, not because punishment is harsh, but because treatments "are the most effective ways of changing outcomes," that is, because they are more effective at eliminating unwanted conduct.[51] To make this clear, the authors begin with an overview of how recent research has transformed our understanding of motivated conduct, in a way that directly challenges the idea that what we do is controlled by an internal calculation of benefits, risks, and consequences.

Addiction research, the authors report, has altered "our understanding of the fundamental biologic processes involved in voluntary behavioral control."[52] (This understanding, we will see, precisely informs the theory and technique of behavioral interventions.) Most importantly, it has transformed how we understand the nature and formation of intention. In the conventional view, our intentions are like inner creations, which we each produce on the basis of a consideration of what we stand to gain and what we stand to lose if we volunteer to undertake a course of action. It turns out, however, that intentions are something *instilled* in us from the outside, as it were, as the result of our encounter with a certain kind of objects. It is a legacy of our biological evolution that certain objects, called *rewards*, can induce the release of dopamine in our brains. When this occurs, a neurological process called "motivational learning" is set in motion. Stimulated by a reward, we *learn* that it is rewarding, and this learning produces a motive, within us, to pursue the object again.[53] This learning is the "fundamental biologic process" that produces intention in a subject, and it is an iterable process: the more one encounters an object, the stronger the motive to pursue it will become. At the subjective level, the strengthening of a motive is experienced as a feeling of *willingness*, of *volition*, to actually seek out the motivating object. "The greater the motivational attribute associated with a reward (e.g., a drug) [that is, the greater one's motive to pursue it, at a biological level] the greater the effort a person is willing to exert and the greater the negative consequences he or she will be willing to endure in order to obtain it."[54] We have, then, this picture of voluntary conduct: an encounter with a reward instills a motive in the brain, which renders us willing to pursue that reward in two ways—willing to *strive* in order to get it, and willing to *suffer* in the course of that striving.

The fact that our intentions are instilled in us by rewarding objects does not mean that we have no capacity for choice. This is because we all encounter a variety of rewards in life, which instill in us a corresponding variety of motives. And where there are competing motives, there is choice.[55] This is why our behavior is not entirely predicted by the history of what we encounter, even though motivational learning is a "fundamental" process of volition in the sense that *all* our motives and modes of willingness are formed by it, whether the willed object is food, friendship, sex, or art.[56] Here, we arrive at a precise understanding of how addiction can form, and what it is. Addiction does not involve abnormal volition; the compulsive pursuit of drugs is secured by "the same molecular mechanisms that strengthen synaptic connections during learning" in all cases of volition.[57] Yet it is a condition in which the capacity for choice is compromised by an absence of sufficient competing motives. This can arise because some objects, like drugs, are so chemically potent that the motives they instill in us (even after just a few encounters) are disproportionately powerful—so strong as to produce a willingness to exert and suffer that is not easily outweighed by other motives. In addiction, "the reward and motivational systems become reoriented to focus on the more potent release of dopamine produced by the drug and its cues," such that "ordinary, healthful rewards lose their former motivational power." The addict is not someone whose willing capacity is broken, but someone whose will pursues just one object, or very few objects. It is as if "the landscape of the person with addiction becomes restricted to one of cues and triggers for drug use."[58] The addict is like a subject in a world barren but for one reward.

With this new understanding of volition and addiction, we are in a position to grasp why behavioral interventions are so promising as an alternative to punishment. If the addict's conduct is not an outcome of impaired volitional capacity or character, it cannot be corrected by punitive means that aim to change such capacity or character. Nor can the addict's conduct be altered by the imposition of suffering. For, as we have seen, the existence of a strongly motivated conduct is evidence of a willingness precisely to endure all kinds of suffering in the performance of that conduct. What is needed, in order to change the conduct of the addict, is a means of intervention that transforms precisely what is wrong with the addict: not the will, not the character, but rather *the restricted land-scape of rewards* that the addict is motivated to pursue. And this calls for more subtle instruments of reform than the conventional techniques of punishment. These are precisely the techniques of behavioral intervention, which promise to achieve what punishment has forever failed to do effectively: not just act humanely, but "improve public safety," "reintegrate [addicts] into society," and "lead to improvements in behavior."[59]

We saw that the power and coherence of TC techniques depended on a particular theory of how the addict comes to differ, in their conduct, from other subjects. The difference at the level of conduct was figured as an epiphenomenal difference, signaling a more basic difference between the development of the addict's will (impaired) and the development of other subjects' will (normal). Hence, TC techniques worked by emulating the conditions under which the will is developed, in order to develop it anew and more normally. Strict confinement, the embrace of a new family, graduated growth, punishment for violating shared values—all these were intended to construct an environment in which the addict's will could once again *grow*, achieving a more mature, non-compulsive, and non-hedonistic quality. By contrast, behavioral interventions draw their power and coherence from the theory of addiction that we have just examined. Here, it is not *maldevelopment of inner will* that explains the addict's conduct, but rather the *instilling of a too-strong motive* in the subject that narrows the range of objects recognized and pursued as rewards. Healing the addict thus consists not in redeveloping or rehabilitating the will, which operates in the same fashion whether one chases one reward or many, but rather in instilling a wider variety of motives in the subject. Such wider variety will enable more flexibility in conduct—as we saw, competing motives enable conscious choice—and thus, a relenting of the addiction. In a word, if the TC sought to reform conduct by rearing the addict, behavioral interventions seek the same by remaking the field of rewards that the subject is exposed to, solicited by, and willing to pursue.

Returning to the *NEJM* article, we learn that behavioral interventions are subdivided into three types of strategy, three ways of pursuing the goal of diversifying the motives instilled in the subject.[60] First, there are "strategies to enhance the salience of natural, healthy rewards such as social contact or exercise [which] could enable those rewards to compete with the direct and acquired motivating properties of drugs."[61] These strategies work by increasing the potency of natural rewards, so that the motives they instill in the subject might become strong enough to compete with the addictive motive. For instance, in contingency management (the first technique advocated in Eldred's brief), healthy rewards such as drug-free socializing or negative drug tests are joined to vouchers, cash prizes, and praise.[62] This gives them bolder presence, as it were, on the previously barren landscape of rewards recognized by the addict, leading them to engage and develop new motives. Second, there are "strategies to help patients recovering from addiction to change their circle of friends and to avoid drug-associated environmental cues." Here, the task is both to surround the subject with novel social rewards and to help the subject avoid contact with the addictive reward. Thus, techniques such as community reinforcement and motivation enhancement therapy (also advocated in Eldred) treat addiction by "improving family relations," facilitating "vocational training," and helping the subject to "develop new recreational activities and social networks."[63] Third, there are "strategies to mitigate a person's stress reactivity . . . and to improve executive function and self-regulation," which can "help recovering patients plan ahead in order to avoid situations in which they are particularly vulnerable to taking drugs." Here again the goal is to reduce contact between the addict and the object of their addiction, and thus to increase the chance that other rewards will solicit the addict. But if the second strategy aims to achieve this by directly arranging the lived contexts of the addict, this third strategy works by shoring up the addict's cognitive capacity to steer themselves away from those settings where addictive objects might be encountered, "developing strategies for coping with cravings and avoiding those high-risk situations"—as in cognitive behavior therapy, the last exemplary method named in Eldred.[64]

Such are the methods that, as we saw in the opening to this chapter, constitute "the most commonly used forms of drug abuse treatment" in our time.[65] And such are the methods that are advocated—on their own, or "assisted" by medications, in MAT—

when the call is made to replace punishment with treatment. This argument for behavioral interventions as an alternative to punishment is made explicitly in the *NEJM* article that we have studied, as well as in *Eldred*, where behavioral interventions are identified as the effective "best practices" in contrast to which the ineffectiveness of punishment is revealed. The same argument is made implicitly by a range of institutional innovations in American criminal justice in our time. To be sure, punishment has not yet fully yielded to treatment as a primary response in the criminal justice system. However, *where* punishment has yielded to treatment, it has most often yielded to behavioral interventions. Consider, for instance, the Law Enforcement Assisted Diversion program, now active in over three-dozen jurisdictions in the United States, which provides police departments with training and resources to bring addicts to city health centers or treatment facilities for "behavioral change" as an alternative to criminal arrest and booking.[66] The same diversion of individuals, from criminal arrest to behavioral therapy, is also now being achieved by the "street crisis response teams" that have emerged as first-line responders to certain 911 calls in many major US cities.[67]

Crucially, what is now becoming common—indeed, a "best practice"—among us in the form of behavioral interventions is more than a newly effective modality of addiction treatment. It is a new approach to reforming human conduct, which can be defined by two features.

First, behavioral interventions involve a distinctive construction of the human. By way of contrast, recall the figure of the human that enabled and structured TC treatment. As we saw, TC treatment was premised on a particular understanding, not just of the addict, but of the subject in general. It presumed that *every* subject is a creature who, under the watch of a family, develops a certain style of willing and acting, and whose natural destiny is to develop a mature way of willing, one that restrains the wild hedonism of infancy and subordinates that early will to pleasure to the pursuit of higher pleasures such as socially productive work, modest and monogamous intimacy, and the building of one's own family. This broad construction of the subject provided an account of addiction—the conduct of the addict was explained by an impaired development of will—and set the aim of addiction treatment—to *re*develop a malformed will. Behavioral interventions, by contrast, figure the subject not as the bearer of a better- or worse-developed character, but as a kind of fertile seedbed for the instillation of motives in response to experiences of reward. In this construction of the human, every subject is presumed to have the same volitional capacities, to develop motives by means of the same molecular processes, and to be susceptible to seduction by the same rewards. What differentiates one individual from the next is not a character, or style of willing, that is set down by early development, but rather the range and flexibility of motives that are active in the subject at this moment, consequent to a certain history of exposure to and engagement with rewards. Thus, the techniques of behavioral intervention can be defined, first, as based on a specific construction of the human subject, which explains addiction as a narrowing of instilled motives and thus sets the target of treatment as an expanded field of motivating rewards.

Second, behavioral interventions can be defined by their distinctive technical apparatus and requirements. Insofar as TC treatment aimed to heal addiction by redeveloping the subject, it had to emulate the structure and instruments of the family, the natural context for development. Thus, TCs had to operate as closed, residential facilities (homes) that sheltered individuals from the dangers and demands of the broader society. And within these facilities, the techniques in use were meant to facilitate intimate surveillance, hierarchical observation, close control of behavior and daily regimen, and the rational dispensation of privileges, punishments, encouragement, and moral admonition. In short, TCs required the technical apparatus of an institution of enclosure, and myriad methods of subjective discipline. By contrast, behavioral interventions are versatile, mobile, and institutionally lean as reformative methods. They do not require a strict organization of peers and staff around members; they do not require any particular architectural or institutional setting; and they do not need to be executed in any particular, let alone carefully graduated and many-months-long, sequence. For what they must emulate is not a process of inner development but rather a process of exposure and instillation that can take place at any time in life, and in any social context. Behavioral interventions, we might say, do not need to embrace and mold the soul and character of the subject. Rather, they simply need to alter the *landscape* around the subject, and seed a new and healthier range of motives in the subject by presenting them with certain rewards and helping them to keep a distance from others. And this can happen without enclosing, closely watching, or controlling the movements of the subject. It can work indirectly, without coercion, and noninvasively; more than an alternative to punishment, behavioral interventions achieve control of conduct by techniques opposed to those of prisons.

We can see, then, how behavioral interventions constitute a technology of reform that is nonetheless compatible with, indeed a vector for, the normalization of addiction. To be sure, the conduct of an addict is unwanted, unhealthy, and unusually compulsive. And yet the *subject* of addiction, and the mechanism of the addict's conduct, are normal. Conduct is to be reformed, not through an alteration of the qualities or characters of the individual, but through expansion of the range of motives that have been instilled at the site of the subject, who is now—was always, will always be—nothing more than a seedbed for the cultivation of motives, hence always vulnerable to the development of addiction. This means that behavioral interventions constitute a technique of power that reforms and transforms conduct, and this in socially decided directions, without a stipulation that the subject on which it acts is deviant, abnormal. Mobile, versatile, institutionally undemanding, indirect, noncoercive, reformative without marking the subject as abnormal—all of these characteristics, taken together, render behavioral interventions legible as a powerful and distinctly *post-disciplinary* technique of power. The rise of behavioral interventions, indeed, may be read as one means for the broader emergence of post-disciplinary powers in our time, a trend that we can now observe within, but which certainly exceeds, the domain of addiction treatment. Let me now develop this last argument further, and more precisely state the link between the rise of behavioral interventions and the larger trend of a move toward post-disciplinary powers. This will be the first of several links forged in this book that allow us to embed the normalization of addiction, starting with its key instances, in a historical-cultural context featuring new or at least newly common ways of constructing and controlling the subject.

As is well known, one of the major touchstones of contemporary social and political theory has been Michel Foucault's characterization of the modern West as a constellation of "disciplinary societies."[68] In a series of works published in the 1970s, Foucault argued that since roughly the eighteenth century, a broad range of central institutions in Euro-Atlantic societies—economic, medical, educational, legal, and more—had increasingly come to rely on disciplinary techniques of power for knowing, evaluating, and reforming the lives of individuals. Foucault's examples of such techniques were varied in their particulars; these examples included the examination and grading of pupils by teachers, the mental and bodily training of infantry by generals, and the use of closely supervised labor as a rehabilitative instrument for prisoners. Yet in all these examples, Foucault spied a consistent method: each person was individually examined and then measured and evaluated in relation to a normative model or ideal type of the human subject (the stellar student, the perfect soldier, the fully reformed prisoner). Failure to approximate the normative model did not always bring down harsh interventions or sanctions, but the method of measuring individuals against an ideal type of the subject increasingly justified and guided interventions and sanctions. Medical profiles, prisoner case histories, student assessments, and worker evaluations, which proliferated in the eighteenth century, were signs of a "disciplinary generalization" in the modern West, a historical tendency for all efforts to reform and improve human life—whether in the hospital, the school, the factory, or the prison—to converge on a single method: the identification of abnormal individuals, and the forced assimilation of such individuals to a normative model of the subject.[69] By the nineteenth century, Foucault argued, there was hardly a venue of life in which subjects were not governed, at one time or another, by such a method of power, which he termed, synthetically, *discipline*.

Foucault's theorization of modern disciplinary societies has inspired countless studies of American society over the last half century. Analyses of disciplinary power in the domains of education, work, and medicine especially abound. Yet, since the early 1990s, Foucault's account has also inspired an important body of scholarship that seeks to trace not the persistence of disciplinary power in contemporary US society, but precisely its faltering in recent times, its waning as a general and pervasive method of subjective reform and control. The earliest widely discussed instance of this thesis emerged in 1992, when Gilles Deleuze proposed that Foucault had illuminated disciplinary power at just the moment when "disciplinary society was what we already no longer were, what we had ceased to be." In this early work, Deleuze did not yet offer a detailed picture of what was to come after the disciplinary society, but nonetheless diagnosed "a generalized crisis in relation to all the environments of enclosure—prison, hospital, factory, school, and family." Deleuze noted "ceaseless" reforms, in the late twentieth century, to render such environments less coercive, less imposing of normative judgments, as if "everyone knows that these institutions are finished" despite not knowing what "new forces [are] knocking at the door."[70] Echoing Deleuze, and focusing on the economic sphere, Nancy Fraser has argued more recently that "Foucault mapped the contours of the disciplinary society just as the ground was being cut out from under it," as flexibilization and deregulation have dissolved the factories and Fordist corporations that once facilitated discipline of workers.[71] In the penal sphere, Malcolm Feeley and Jonathan Simon have argued that although prisons have certainly not been dissolved in American society, since the 1970s there has been an important shift in the rationality of their use: a move away "from a concern with reforming the individual to managing segments of the 'population,'" or a displacement of disciplinary by actuarial concerns.[72] And in a broader study of contemporary American social life, Bernard Harcourt suggests that there is "little need today to discipline us. We are no longer forced to follow strict timetables and work routines, to walk in straight lines, stand at attention, or stay seated behind rows of school desks. No need to confine us to observation and examination."[73] For today we no longer need to be deeply and intimately observed to be identified as individuals and to have our conduct directed. The information that we constantly shed as users of digital systems may not reveal us as full persons, and yet it reveals our interests, opinions, and preferences enough to facilitate control through targeted ads, nudges, recommendations, and selective presentation of choice. The point variously made by these authors is not that discipline is fully finished and over, but that a new trend is legible in late-modern US society: the invention and growing prominence of new techniques of control that are non-disciplinary and non-repressive in method, and even figured as repudiations of and advances on disciplinary methods.

Each of these authors theorizes, in their own way, the emergence of such new methods of control. Deleuze, at the most general level, characterizes the new forces at the door as techniques for shaping conduct through constant competition, comparison, and mutual adjustment among institutions and partial attributes of persons, without reference to any ideal outcome or normative model of the individual.[74] Fraser describes the increasing use of "flexible, fluctuating networks" to organize production, joined with the evaluation of individuals not in relation to an ideal norm but as bearers of human-capital value, as the dominant techniques of economic power in a "post-disciplinary society."[75] Feeley and Simon propose that the method of "population management," "rather than social or personal transformation," informs the "emerging strategy of corrections."[76] Harcourt offers "expository power" as a name for the new methods of control enabled by bits of information passively shed by users, which are increasingly eliminating any need for the kinds of deep surveillance, examination, and evaluation facilitated by disciplinary methods.[77]

Let us situate our study of behavioral interventions in the context of these other analyses. My claim is that behavioral interventions merit consideration, alongside flexibilized networks of production and the capitalization of workers, risk-oriented and population-managing punishment, and exposition and coordination of users on digital platforms, as a distinct and potent method of power that facilitates control over conduct by non-repressive, post-disciplinary means. They thus merit consideration, as well, as a vector and reflection of the larger trend established by all these new methods of power: the decreasing reliance on discipline as a technique for reforming conduct in late-modern American society and the knocking of new forces at our door.

Behavioral interventions constitute a *post-disciplinary* method of power in three ways. Like disciplinary power, behavioral interventions are clearly aimed at transforming the conduct of the individual in the name of the social, and not only personal, interest. As we saw, behavioral interventions promise to supersede punishment as the most effective means of advancing public safety, social integration, and improvement of conduct at the site of addicted subjects. And yet behavioral interventions achieve these aims, first, without figuring conduct as an expression of *individuality*. Indeed, the individual as such never appears in the course of behavioral therapy. Contrast this with TC treatment, in the course of which addictive acts are read as the expression of a deformed character and an underdeveloped volitional capacity, and in which the addict's status as an individual is clearly marked and positioned within a graduated hierarchy of maturity. In the TC, the placement of each individual at a stage in the temporal progression of treatment and at a stratum in the pyramidal social structure of the facility enabled a precise measurement of the distance that remained between each member and the model form of the human that they were meant to achieve. In behavioral interventions, there is no comparison of the individual with any other, let alone with an ideal subject; there is only a measure of the number and flexibility of the motives presently active in the subject and a mapping of the subject's environs.

Second, behavioral interventions, like other post-disciplinary methods of power, control conduct without directly targeting, coercing, or molding the body of the individual. Whereas in the TC, constant regulation of movement and daily activity, restraints on disruptive conduct and expression, and surveillance for conformity to facility codes and values are essential instruments of treatment, behavioral interventions require no institutional confinement and no direct limits on the movements of the body. As we saw, behavioral interventions do not manipulate the body; they manipulate the landscape of rewards by which the body is surrounded, and at most, equip the subject with cognitive-behavioral strategies for reshaping that landscape themselves. There is no place or use for direct coercion, and only exposure of the body to healthier rewards and their solicitations. Presenting these healthier rewards, combined with clearing away unhealthy objects, is enough to alter the conduct of the subject; the normal mechanisms of learning and volition in the subject, once presented with these healthier rewards, take care of the rest.

And third, behavioral interventions are post-disciplinary in their invention of a new sense of the *norm* that ought to regulate and adjust individual conduct. In TCs, the operative norm is a normative model of character or personality, an ideal figure of the individual that is embodied by the more advanced members, imperfectly, and by the staff-parents, more perfectly. Indeed, in the TC a crucial method of treatment is *identification* with these more perfect individuals; the addict is healed to the extent that they internalize a normative model of the subject and gradually materialize that model as the shape and essence of their own body. In behavioral interventions, there is a norm that governs the reform of conduct, but this is not a figure of ideal individuality. It is narrower and more underdetermined than such an ideal figure of the subject. It consists only in a certain *range* and *flexibility* of motives animating the conduct of the individual, while making no judgment about character, essence, or personality. In fact, the norm of conduct for behavioral interventions does not even discriminate against the object of addiction; after all, what renders the drug an unhealthy or unnatural reward is simply its extreme potency, and not its status as morally objectionable, unproductive, or cheap. What is abnormal in addiction is neither the subject nor the object, but only the number and strength of rewards soliciting the conduct of the subject at this moment. And the norm of health is not strict abstinence, or an indifference to the appeal of hedonistic objects, like drugs, but rather a modicum of choice enabled by a range of competing motives.

All three characteristics—the elision of the individual, the indirection of their techniques, and the reproduction of a norm that regulates range, not quality—allow for the improvement of conduct without any of the moralizing judgment, intimate control, or institutional burdens that attend discipline. And yet, let us remember, behavioral interventions promise to realize what the prison could never effectively achieve: the elimination of unwanted conduct, and thus the goods of offender reintegration, social order, and public safety. Thus, behavioral interventions represent not an abdication of regulatory ambitions, but a way of realizing them without use of disciplinary techniques. In this precise sense, they compose a *post-disciplinary* technology of power. To be clear, I am not here casting behavioral interventions as the actualization of a preexisting type. Nor am I suggesting that they have been directly modeled on techniques that have been developed in the domains of work, punishment, digital profiling, and elsewhere in the last forty years. And yet, even as I do not see the rise of behavioral interventions as a simple or direct effect of the rise of post-disciplinary power, I do see it as importantly *enabled* by the latter, and perhaps more importantly, as itself a *furthering* of the move beyond discipline as a dominant mode of power in the late-modern United States. Let me conclude this discussion by developing these richer relationships between behavioral interventions and post-disciplinary power, which appear differently depending on how the condition of a post-disciplinary society is conceived.

If it is true, as Deleuze, Fraser, Harcourt, and others argue, that discipline is waning as a dominant mode of power in American society, we might conceive the present moment, first, as one without a dominant mode of power, characterized instead by a discordant multiplicity of ways of constructing and governing subjects. This is how Fraser, for instance, seems to conceive post-disciplinary society. She writes that even though we can try "to identify the characteristic ordering mechanisms and political rationality of the emerging new mode of regulation," we have to recognize that whatever this mode is, it is characterized by "considerable dispersion"; indeed, it may not make sense to speak of a single mode of regulation or governance at all. Or, if we do speak of a single mode, we might need to conceive it as a "ruling apparatus whose composition is so complex and shifting that [some have] named it '*la nébuleuse*.'"[78] If we accept this picture of post-disciplinary society, we can read the place of the rise of behavioral interventions within it in two ways. First, as a phenomenon *conditioned* by the new multiplicity of powers, and the fall of discipline's hegemony. Insofar as behavioral interventions, as we have seen, not only make no use of disciplinary figures and methods, but explicitly disavow such figures and methods as cruel and ineffective, the waning of discipline's broad acceptance as a cultural commonplace certainly constitutes a crucial condition, a clearing of the ground, for the rise of behavioral intervention as a noncontroversial, mainstream, and locally dominant form of treatment. And second, insofar as behavioral interventions constitute, again, a challenge to and even *replacement* for discipline, at least within one important domain of conduct reform and treatment, it clearly furthers the waning of discipline as a commonplace and conventional set of techniques, undermining the latter both in practice and in theory.

A second view of our present is, of course, that the waning of discipline is followed by, or simultaneous with, the rise of a new dominant power modality in our society. In this view, the condition of post-disciplinary power has a positive, and not simply negative, meaning; it refers not just to the proliferation of *non-disciplinary* powers, but to the emergence of a distinct modality of power that can be called post-disciplinary. Several of our post-disciplinary theorists propose this kind of view. Deleuze predicted, for instance, "the progressive and dispersed installation of a new system of domination." Feeley and Simon speak of "*the* new penology" that "increasingly shapes the way the power to punish is exercised" in American late modernity. Harcourt heralds, boldly, "the birth of the expository society."[79] Of course, as yet, none of these proposals, which have been influential in their own fields, has managed to capture a truly general mode of power such as discipline, revealing and encompassing a distinctive approach to control at work across domains including health, education, criminal justice, economy, and more. But this should not surprise us, since the works of Deleuze, Feeley, Simon, and Harcourt represent efforts to theorize a new dominant power modality at the very beginning of its emergence, without the long view that Foucault could take on discipline two centuries after its birth. It is worth remembering here why, in Foucault's account, disciplinary power itself took so long to fully emerge. In *Discipline and Punish*, Foucault writes that discipline as a dominant modality of power was not the result of an "invention," not consequent to a "sudden discovery." Rather, the rise to dominance or what Foucault called the "generalization" of discipline in Western societies began in "a multiplicity of often minor processes, of different origin and scattered location."[80] It began, that is, with a local innovation in monastic procedures here, a development of a new way of managing workers there, and so forth. Only over time were these scattered methods "combined and generalized" to form a unified technique of discipline, both in thought (through abstract reflections on the optimal use of power, such as in Bentham's Panopticon studies) and in practice (through institutional projects that joined, say, the power of psychologists and teachers in schools, or physicians and bosses in factories, which facilitated mutual exchange and reinforcement of their techniques).[81] So the rise of a dominant modality of power takes time, because it requires the independent development of a variety of techniques, which can then be combined and generalized to form a broad method of power that can be widely applied and rendered consistent in society. Crucially, however, not just any scattered methods can be combined and generalized. Rather, what allowed the techniques that would become discipline to come together was their rough isomorphism and strategic similarity: their shared concern, disparately developed, with evaluating individuals at a deep, personal level and with bringing these individuals into line with an ideal model of the human personality, whether in the language and for the sake of religious salvation, mental health, or education. Perhaps we are in a time *between* the emergence of scattered, isomorphic techniques and their combination into a new dominant mode of power. If so, we might see the rise of behavioral interventions in the domain of addiction treatment not just as a development enabled by the waning of discipline as a hegemonic mode, and not just as a contributor to that waning, but also as the rise of a technique that, with its resemblance to a host of other techniques of power that have developed in the last forty years as advances beyond discipline, may become one ingredient for the development of a broader, generalized modality of power ascendant in our near future. After all, as we have seen, there is a striking concordance between behavioral interventions and other post-disciplinary powers in our time, on at least the following features: elision of the individual underlying conduct; a leanness and mobility in its technical apparatus; and use of gentle and indirect inducements to change the acts, but only the acts, of the evaluated and governed subject. Perhaps behavioral interventions are one means by which a new dominant mode of power to come is emerging, not in miniature, but in a multiplicity of scattered yet combinable techniques, in our time.

Less than fully causal, but more than mere similarity, the relationships between the rise of behavioral interventions and the rise of other post-disciplinary powers, or indeed the rise of post-disciplinary power as a condition of late-modern American society, constitute our first rich set of links between an instance of the normalization of addiction and the broader historical-cultural context of its appearance. The rise of behavioral interventions constitutes a technique of power that reforms conduct without targeting the abnormality of the individual; in doing so, it enables, finds support in, and perhaps even joins with, a number of other developments generating post-disciplinary powers in late-modern American society. Neither the specific case nor the broader cultural trend, of course, fully explains or comprehends the other. Yet each specifies and throws light upon the other: the rise of behavioral interventions provides the move beyond disciplinary power with concrete illustration and empirical location, while the thesis of post-discipline helps us to see what is conditioning and furthered by our case of normalization. In chapters to come I continue with the effort to spark mutual light between the normalizations of addiction and the social terrain on which they have occurred, but with different relationships in view: between the recent reimagination of addictive craving and a broader reshaping of human desire, in the next chapter, and between the proliferation of addiction discourse since the 1970s and the spread of a new mode of self-relation, in the fourth.

One clarification is needed before moving forward. Foucault, of course, gave us not only the analysis of disciplinary society, but the very project of tracing shifts in dominant modalities of power, at least of the kind pursued here. One issue he never settled, however, was precisely how to understand the *dominance* of a given power modality. He certainly broached the issue on several occasions. For instance, in his 1978 lectures, Foucault himself hypothesized the waning of discipline as a dominant modality of power in his own time, and outlined the rise of a new modality that he called "security." This was not a revision of his analysis of modern society as suffused by disciplinary powers, but rather an extension of that analysis. He wanted to chart what he called a passage from "the modern system" to the "contemporary system," a move beyond disciplinary dominance in the late twentieth century.[82] But he did not want to cast this move as a replacement of one totality by another. The history of modalities of power, he wrote, "is not a series of successive elements, the appearance of the new causing the earlier ones to disappear." Rather, "what above all changes is the dominant characteristic, or more exactly, the system of correlation" of different forms of power in a society. What changes is the *hierarchy* of powers in a society. A dominant power modality is thus not an *exclusive* one, but rather one that is *superordinate* in the sense of being (1) actively promoted (the project of expanding it is a "fundamental question," a social priority); (2) broadly perceived as justified (it causes minimal "scandal" or "friction"); and (3) widely instanced (or "multiplied"). The passing of discipline as a dominant power would thus entail not its disappearance, but rather the waning of its social legitimacy and its withdrawal from crucial contexts. Some forms of discipline will persist in a post-disciplinary society; after all, "things do not necessarily develop in step in different sectors, at a given moment, in a given society, in a given country."[83]

Foucault's qualification here is crucial, but insufficient. Recent scholars working within and beyond the Foucauldian frame have taken his acknowledgment of social unevenness, or the disparate development of power in different sectors of society, a step further. They point out that the uneven development of modalities of power in a society is not random or infinitely complex. Rather, it falls along obvious lines of social difference. We know that class, gender, and race are not just identity markers. They are determinants, or at least predictors, of the forms of power to which any given person is likely to be exposed. What is more, we know that *subordinate* class, gender, and racial status is a reliable predictor of exposure to unjustified power, patently brutal power, that is, forms of power that others in society would perceive as cruel, because outmoded. In fact, it may be that subjection, routinely and still, to modalities of power that no longer enjoy wide social acceptance and legitimacy, or that are at least no longer applied to the superordinate classes of society, who are governed by more progressive, more accepted forms of power—it may be that subjection to scandalous and subordinate powers, to use Foucault's terminology, is part of what constitutes subordinate positions of race, gender, and class within a society.

I think here, for instance, of a recent essay by the cultural theorist Grant Farred, in which he reads the 2022 racist massacre at Masten Park as revealing, in part, the particular subjection suffered by poorer Black Americans in our day. Farred begins by affirming Foucault's narrative of a shift, in the course of modernity, from sovereignty to biopolitics as the dominant modality of population governance. This helps Farred to explain how the Masten Park shooter could expect to find so many Black victims at the Tops supermarket he targeted. In the age of biopolitics, the movement of bodies is controlled, Farred argues, not by fiat or force but by the orchestration of choice. And because Masten Park is a food desert, with just one grocery store within accessible distance, its Black residents are induced, even as they decide, to gather at the Tops supermarket. But as soon as the point is made, Farred finds the analysis wanting. For what is so glaring in the Masten Park massacre is the extent to which the residents there are not simply governed through their choices, but also "subject to a power that decides on who lives and who dies"—subject, that is, to sovereign violence, although in the form of vigilante violence enabled (through withdrawal of police protection from the Masten Park community, considered unworthy of such protection) rather than directly exercised by the state. What the massacre at Masten Park reveals is that if we now live in the age of biopolitics, then "in the age of biopolitics, black and minority life remains uniquely vulnerable to . . . sovereign violence." Indeed, Farred goes so far as to suggest that this vexed historical condition, this subjection to sovereign violence in the age of its delegitimation, partly defines the social position of Masten Park residents in our day. The "contradiction" of sovereign subjection in a biopolitical age "mark[s] that demographic point where biopolitics and sovereignty each reveal their own benefits," where "black residents of Buffalo's East side are made victim to each."[84]

Farred's analysis yields two crucial lessons about the project of tracing shifts in dominant modalities of power. The first is that such a project is, on its own, incomplete. If the ultimate aim is to cast light on how power works in our society, then the analysis of a newly dominant power has to be extended and qualified by a study of how it is realized differently in different sectors of society, that is, for different demographics, different positions of class, gender, race, and so forth. At the same time, Farred's analysis suggests that tracing shifts in dominant modalities of power can actually help us to articulate demographic differences, and to understand how certain racial, gender, and class positions are socially produced as subordinate. What if part of that production happens precisely through the subjection of some demographic groups, but not others, to forms of power that are patently no longer dominant—that is, no longer theoretically justified, common, and widespread, let alone considered progressive? What if the subordination and even the very distinctiveness of a demographic position were maintained, that is, by its subjection to forms of power understood as primitive and outmoded? Perhaps, to stay with Farred's example, it is not just because the Masten Park residents are Black or poor that they are subjected to sovereign violence amid a biopolitical age; perhaps that subjection is also, in part, what produces those residents as apart and different from those in whiter and richer communities.

Or, to come back to our analysis: it is certain that the shift in power modalities charted in this chapter is unevenly realized in late-modern American society. That there has been a broad shift, *within* the domain of treatment, toward the use of behavioral interventions and away from disciplinary techniques is clear. But access to treatment is dependent on race, class, gender, and geography in complex ways.[85] And this means that the post-disciplinary governance of addiction is farther advanced for certain demographic groups in our society than others: for those who live in cities rather than rural areas; for those who can afford to attend and stay in treatment; for those in the criminal justice system most likely to be diverted to treatment, that is, whites; and so forth. Indeed, it may be that governance by post-disciplinary power as opposed to control by arrest and confinement constitutes one form of contemporary superordination in our society (as paradoxical as it may be to identify superordination in subjection).[86] If so, then the project of studying a shift toward post-disciplinary powers in late-modern American society is not at odds with the task of illuminating the unevenness of this shift in reality; it invites and supports the second task, and finds fulfillment in it. In this book I am generally focused on the broad cultural changes revealed by the normalization of addiction, what I describe as shifts in dominant modes of subject-construction in late-modern American society. I take this focus, not because I consider it sufficient or complete, but because the broad trends are what my material has led me to see most clearly. And I do so with the hope that illuminating the broad trends can serve two ends simultaneously: to help us see the large movements now transforming our understandings of the subject, and to help us see, as well, the difference of those social places where these movements fail, in part or fully, to reach.

Measuring Our Desire
Craving, Therapy, Tracking, Rating

This chapter examines yet another case of the normalization of addiction in late-modern American society. This is the emergence of a novel scientific theory of addictive craving in the early 1990s, which is now often presented as a standard explanation for craving in both scientific literature and public media. According to this theory, the craving of the addict is not a unique modality of desire but rather the quantitative maximum of desire, which only ever exists in a single modality. The significance of this theory of craving lies not only in its normalization of addiction but in its reimagination of *all* human desire such that addictive craving can appear simply as intense desire, desire that is unduly strong, yet normal and familiar in its development and quality. The new theory of craving, as we will see, casts all human desire as a kind of amassed quantity in the subject that is produced in the subject by an attractive object, and as an impulse whose strength is determined primarily by the qualities of the object—by the absolute attractiveness of the object—rather than by the inner life or character of the desiring body and mind. In recasting human desire in this way, the new theory of craving now circulating in a wide variety of texts on addiction appears to reflect and amplify a certain tendency in late-modern US culture: a tendency to figure human desire as a measurable quantity, as a kind of literal motion, and as determined in the main by the potency of the desired object, which we will find in a range of recent developments, including the rise of cognitive behavior therapy, the rise of self-tracking as a popular activity, and the naturalization of ratings as a measure of desirability.

In order to grasp the emergence of a new figure of desire in all these developments as a *recasting* or *re*imagination of desire, we first need a clear picture of the alternative figure of desire that the new figure excludes and succeeds. For much of the twentieth century, in venues ranging from medical science to policy debates, addiction was often conceived as the result of a regression of the subject into a primitive psychic condition, a condition whose core feature is an indiscriminate, uncontrolled, and base modality of desire.[1] One exemplary instance of this view can be found in a scholarly monograph on addiction published by a medical press in the mid-1980s and authored by the physician and US drug czar Ian Macdonald. There we read that "chemical dependency," that is, addiction, is best understood by analogy to "natural dependency," by which Macdonald means the psychic state of a child.[2] Both are defined by a certain type of desire: pursuit of "euphoria," inability to submit that pursuit to the constraints of reality ("distorted reality testing"), a tendency to act immediately on hedonistic motive ("impulsiv[ity]"), and incapacity to deal with frustration of desire ("lack [of] the tools necessary for dealing with stress and intimacy").[3] In fact, addiction and psychic immaturity are more than analogous; addiction *is* regression to an immature psychic state: "the 18-year-old chemically dependent child may be seen as delinquent (which he is) or as depressed (which he is), or he may be seen as a 13-year-old."[4] The addict is a pseudo-adult, who desires like a child—crudely, incessantly—despite having developed physically: "an 'adult' who is amoral and without an ethical code except as it relates to personal desire."[5]

Significant here is not just the claim that addiction is akin to immaturity, and that what makes addiction abnormal is its primitive quality. More crucial is the broader understanding of desire that supports an analysis of addiction as regression to the pleasure-life of early childhood or infancy. This is an understanding of desire as a kind of errant force in the subject that pushes the body toward any and all sites of pleasure, yet also a force that can be refined into more stable and mature forms of attachment and intimacy. This is, of course, an understanding of desire that was consecrated in the language of psychoanalysis and ego psychology. Thus, Macdonald cites Freud and Erik Erikson to lay the ground for his study of addiction: we know, he presumes, that "man by nature seeks pleasure," but that with maturation the drive to pleasure is normally sublimated into "industry" and "achievement," regulated and moderated by an "ethical code," and channeled by "heterosexual identification."[6] It was this broader understanding of desire as a force capable of being refined through sublimation and social regulation that enabled addictive craving, that is, the uncontrolled pursuit of drug use and its pleasures, to be conceived as a primitive or untrammeled modality of desire, as desire set loose, run wild, and regressed to an immature, even animalistic, kind and quality. And it was this understanding of desire that structured the forms of treatment most popular in the middle third of the twentieth century—often, psychoanalytically informed therapy for those who could afford private clinical treatment, or the maturation program of therapeutic communities—as well as the forms of punishment applied to those deemed unworthy or incapable of being healed by treatment: exclusion (by imprisonment) from a society whose demands of psychic maturity and civilized desire the regressed addict could no longer meet.

Thus, the background understanding of desire, and of the desiring subject, that enabled twentieth-century constructions of addiction as primitive desire was what Foucault, in *The History of Sexuality, Volume One*, theorized as the *confessional* figure of desire. Foucault, of course, argued that the confessional figure of desire found its culmination in the theory and practice of psychoanalysis, where desire was explicitly constructed as a personal drive lurking in the depths of the subject that could be revealed through verbal confession, like a secret. But he found this figure, first, in his analysis of the scientific and medical discourses on sex that emerged in the early and mid-nineteenth century, which also constituted sexual desire as a hidden personal drive that determines the life and acts of the body. And in studying the history of the modern sexual sciences, Foucault found further that the confessional construction of desire in fact went far beyond the domain of erudite knowledge about sexuality. As is well known, Foucault's study of sexual science led him to see the modern West as "a singularly confessing society," by which he meant a society in which the confession of desire was performed and expected in a wide range of cultural venues, and in which desire was thus widely construed as the sort of thing that can be confessed. Foucault saw the confessional figure of desire in the moral-theological discourses, the judicial practices, and the educational institutions of eighteenth- and nineteenth-century Western societies: in this period, he argued, Catholic penance became newly focused on oral confession of the "impulses" or "stirrings" of the soul; judges increasingly pressed criminals to speak not just of their acts, but of their deep asocial instincts and tendencies; and ordinary students were increasingly surveilled for signs of sexual interest and awakening. Hence, Foucault argued that the confessional figure of desire, far from the invention of psychoanalysis, or even of the modern sciences of sexuality, was a conventional and general framework for desire in the modern West, an understanding of desire that was codified in, but that also far exceeded, the analysis of libido and unconscious instinct in the various sciences of sexuality.

I draw on Foucault's analysis of confessional desire to frame the work of this chapter in two ways. First, the figure of confessional desire precisely captures the basic understanding of desire that underlay constructions of addictive craving as primitive desire in many twentieth-century accounts of addiction. It helps us to describe and portray what desire was imagined to be, such that craving could appear as a regressed or broken-down desire. And this will help us to see clearly what is displaced and challenged by the new scientific theory of craving as the maximum of normal desire. The creators of this theory themselves presented it as a repudiation of the understanding of desire they saw as most prominent in twentieth-century American addiction science, one that cast desire as a drive to pleasure, and craving as the drive to pleasure let loose or run wild. Analyzing that earlier prominent understanding as an instance of confessional desire will help us to articulate what exactly is set aside and challenged through the normalization of craving, and what new figure, not just of desire but of the desiring subject, is produced in that process. Second, Foucault's analysis of confessional desire will help us to grasp the importance of the reimagination of desire achieved by the normalization of craving. If the confessional figure of desire was not just a rare local thesis, but a conventional, even dominant, construction of desire in the modern West, then its repudiation by the new theory of craving appears as a challenge to a modern cultural convention and not merely a quarrel with an isolated scientific theory. This raises the possibility of comparison. That is, such a reading of the reimagination of desire in the new science of craving allows us to ask: are there other places in our society where the confessional figure of desire had been conventional, but has been challenged in a deep way over the last forty years? Is the repudiation of the modern convention of constructing desire on a confessional model restricted to the normalization of craving? Or is it also instanced elsewhere, in other domains, and achieved by other theories and practices in our time?

In fact, this chapter finds not only that this challenge is widely occurring in late-modern American society, but also that this challenge now appears to be taking a certain consistent form. To make this case, I first offer a conceptual account of the challenge posed to the confessional figure of desire by the neuroscientific theory of incentive-salience attribution, which is now often presented as the leading account of addictive craving.[7] This theory explicitly crafts a novel figure of desire, according to which desire is not an inner drive that is progressively refined through psychic maturation, but a discrete sensitivity and attraction to an alluring object that is formed through encounters with, and enjoyment of, that object at any point in the subject's life. Desire is thus not a quality of the subject, or at least not an abiding one. It is something that is formed in the subject, but that is not, as it were, of the subject. It exists in the subject because of the object that one has encountered, and its strength and target are reflections, not of how far the subject's maturation has proceeded, but rather of the potency of the object that has stimulated the subject. This means that desire cannot be interpreted as a sign of the subject's soul, character, or psyche. The presence of desire in the subject is only a sign that they have enjoyed an attractive object, enjoyment of which would instill desire in any subject alike. Nor is the presence of one desire predictive of any other desire, since each desire is formed in the subject discretely. (When desire was read as a sign of psychic maturity, or character quality, the presence of one primitive desire could indicate the presence of others—hence, addictive craving was frequently said to be predictive of sexual perversion and criminal impulse.[8]) Finally, because desire is not, according to the new figure, a sign of personal quality or a unitary drive deep within the self, it is not a secret to be confessed, or something to be read for symbolic meaning. Rather, it is a measurable quantity, a literal and discrete attraction between an object and the self, and hence something to be tracked and numerically registered, not revealed in self-disclosive language.

In what follows, I will describe the different aspects of this new figure of desire discretely and in detail. But I will also sometimes refer to the rethinking of desire achieved by this new figure as a "de-confessionalization" of desire, as a shorthand. In the next section of this chapter, I explain how the process of de-confessionalization is achieved in the new theory of addictive craving, which renders craving as the quantitative maximum of normal desire, and thus as a paradigm of desire. I then examine three other historical developments that occurred contemporaneously with the emergence and broadening acceptance of the new theory of craving. These other developments are, superficially, unrelated to the normalization of addictive craving. But I will reveal them as three other means by which the de-confessionalization of desire has occurred in the last forty years. In the emergence of cognitive behavior therapy and the waning of psychoanalysis as dominant forms of psychotherapy, in the rise of self-tracking as an increasingly popular method of self-examination, and in the dissemination of the rating as a natural metric for the attractiveness (or what is sometimes called the "desirability") of objects, we will find that desire has been de-confessionalized in these crucial and consistent ways: figured (1) as captured best by quantitative metrics and poorly by expressive language; (2) as revealing the potency and quality of objects rather than the identity and personality of the one who desires; and (3) as originating not in the subject, but out there, in the objects that attract us.

My argument here is not, of course, that the de-confessionalized figure of desire that has emerged across these four developments in addiction science, psychotherapy, self-examination, and evaluative culture represents the only way of understanding desire in our time, or even the hegemonic construction of desire presented to us from all sides in late-modern American society. My argument is, however, a slightly more modest version of that too-ambitious claim. I see the de-confessionalized figure of desire, and of the desiring subject, as an ascendant framework for the experience of desire, and of the self that desires, in our historical time and place. Just as the confessional figure of the subject became a familiar and widely instanced, even in some contexts naturalized, way of making sense of the experience of desire in the modern West, it may well be that a de-confessionalized—a metricized, de-personalized, and object-induced—figure of desire is becoming ever more common as it is carried and reinforced in a growing range of cultural sites and developments in our time. My hope is to offer, starting from an analysis of the construction of desire in contemporary addiction science, a *prism*, similar in concept but not content to the one that Foucault gave us, for seeing how desire is increasingly understood, in reflections on addiction but also elsewhere, in late-modern American society.

Across a wide range of scholarly, government, and popular venues, addiction is now recognized to involve a form of brain disease. Indeed, the neuroscience of addiction is cited as the standard medical view on addiction in most relevant public-oriented productions in this country, including the recent landmark Surgeon General's Report on addiction (and numerous other publications by state agencies over the past few decades) and the 2007 Emmy-winning HBO documentary, likely still the most-watched film of its kind, titled *Addiction*. Importantly, the neuroscientific model of addiction understands it not as a discrete pathological state that begins at a single moment—as in the model of a viral infection that marks the causal and temporal origin of the disease—but rather as a set of interrelated processes, which usually develop in the course of three sequential stages.[9] This matters, for our purposes, because the scientific model of addiction comprises both the stage in which an intense desire to use drugs (or to engage in another addictive behavior) first emerges and a later pair of stages in which developments in several other brain regions unrelated to desire tend to *reinforce* the addictive craving (put simply, the massive release of dopamine within the limbic system of the brain, which mediates desire, induces homeostatic responses whose effects are "between-system" and not only "within-system"—leading, for instance, to heightened stress responses in the amygdala that indirectly contribute to the desirous motivation to use drugs[10]). In what follows, I will be focused on the development of craving, the first stage of addiction, alone, for it is here that *desire*—as opposed to the full variety of brain adaptations that result from long-term substance use (or again, another addictive behavior) and reinforced craving—is centrally at issue. In particular, I want to examine the theory of incentive-salience attribution, which is now widely accepted, or at least presented, as an authoritative account of this desire-forming stage.[11]

The theory of incentive-salience attribution was introduced by the neuroscientists Terry Robinson and Kent Berridge in 1993.[12] It was intended, according to the authors, to replace what were then the conventional answers to what they call "the question of addiction"—namely, why addicts cannot cease their addictive behavior—all of which reflected a deep confusion about the nature of addictive desire.[13] The first, and most traditional, answer was that addicts are driven by a uniquely intense desire for pleasure—they return to the drug because they so powerfully want the euphoria that the drug promises. The second answer, an inverse of the first, was that addicts are driven by their desire to relieve pain—in particular, the pains of withdrawal consequent to chronic drug use. The third answer was not quite an answer, but a popular position nonetheless: many scholars writing at the same time as Robinson and Berridge, they suggest, had accepted the theoretical outlook of B. F. Skinner and simply refused the question of *why* addicts act as they do. These scholars thus simply defined drugs as positive reinforcers and sought to ascertain the environmental conditions under which reinforcement by drugs is more or less successful; on their view, it was sufficient to say that "people take drugs . . . because drugs promote drug-taking behavior"—a premise that gave rise to a great deal of effective experimental research, but which was theoretically vacuous.[14]

To the extent that the question of addiction still mattered, the behaviorist solution could be rejected as empty. But the first two answers had to be rejected as well, this time on the basis of empirical fact. A great deal of experimental research had shown that craving tends to intensify over the course of an addiction, even though the pleasures of drug use reliably wane over time, consequent to the development of tolerance. Further, research had shown that addictive cravings are often felt most intensely when withdrawal symptoms are weakest (just before and during drug use), and that many drugs (like cocaine) have no withdrawal effects yet are clearly highly addictive.[15] Hence, the idea that addictive desire is a drive to pursue euphoric pleasure or a drive to avoid pain could no longer be supported.

In their own research, Robinson and Berridge found that the failure of the conventional responses to the question of addiction could be traced to a misconstrual of how desire develops in the brain, and how it manifests psychologically thereafter. The problem was not an undue focus on subjective desire (as the Skinnerian behaviorists claimed) but rather the unjustified and long-standing presumption that desire is bound up with, if not determined by, experiences of pleasure and pain—that desire is always a desire *for* pleasure or, what is the same, a desire to escape pain. What if the manifest divergence of craving and pleasure, craving and pain, in the case of addiction were an indication that desire and pleasure are only contingently related, converging at times but naming two entirely discrete neurological and psychic experiences? What if desire, if not always then at least sometimes, developed with no reference to pleasure at all?

These are precisely the conclusions at which Robinson and Berridge arrived through their work on the mesolimbic dopamine system, long known to be the brain region directly targeted by drugs and other addictive objects, and long assumed (by scholars and the public alike) to be the site where pleasure is mediated in the brain. Contrary to that long-standing assumption, Robinson and Berridge found that pleasure responses cannot be reliably affected through experimental manipulation of the mesolimbic circuits.[16] Here, pleasure, or what Robinson and Berridge term "liking," refers to the experience of "positive affective states"[17]—it is the feeling that washes over the subject in the wake of a dose of sugar, or in the moment of a thrilling touch. Crucially, Robinson and Berridge found further that experimental manipulation of the mesolimbic system did reliably affect something else, namely, "wanting," or the psychological experience of desire. In other words, they found that the mesolimbic system facilitates the development, within the subject, of *a psychic and bodily inclination toward certain objects*, an inclination that may well overlap with an expectation of pleasure or good feeling, but which is not driven by or invariably tied to such an expectation. And having observed this phenomenological distinction between desire, on the one hand, and pleasure, on the other, they set out to describe, in an independent manner, how it is that desire develops in the subject when real objects stimulate the mesolimbic circuits, and what, if not a drive to pursue pleasure, desire really is.

In a phrase, their theory is that "the psychological process that leads to 'wanting'"—in other words, the formation of desire— "involves the attribution of attractive salience to stimuli and their representations."[18] *Attribution* is a term of art here, and its crucial meaning can be made clear through a comparison to the psychoanalytic notion of *projection*. In projection, the subject *sends* or *throws out* a meaning or image that is primarily formed within the psyche of the subject: the object is endowed with a value or sense that is the subject's own. If my desire for the object involves my projection onto the object, then what I want in the object is at least in part my own making, and this means that my desire is *personal*, inflected and informed by who I am and how my psyche construes the object world. By contrast, attribution is a process in which the subject does not *invest* the object with a personalized value or meaning, but rather *registers* the potency of the stimulating object within its neural circuits and perceptual field. The degree to which the potency of the object is registered may vary according to the conditions under which the subject encounters the object, but the potency itself is determined, first and foremost, by the features of the object itself and their capacity to stimulate neurotransmitter activity in the reward circuits of the subject's brain. In this sense, attribution might be said to reverse the vector of projection, such that desire is formed when the *object's* features are impressed upon the subject. Here is how the process unfolds, in temporal sequence:

To say that attribution reverses the vector of projection is not to suggest that the object is the causal origin of desire in a comprehensive sense. Yet it is to suggest that we can no longer locate that causal origin fully within the subject. According to the theory of attribution, desire begins in the encounter between subject and object, or in the moment when the object stimulates the subject. This moment may well be voluntarily arranged by the subject, but it might just as well be imposed on the subject, by accident or fully against the subject's will; in most cases, the encounter between subject and object is the result of a complex range of factors, including but not reducible to the voluntary choice of the subject.[19] In any case, incentive-salience attribution begins when an object that is capable of inducing desire (that is, of stimulating dopamine release in the mesolimbic circuits of the brain) stimulates the subject "via sensory receptors" (tongue, skin, eyes, etc.) or "more directly" (by ingestion, injection, or electric brain stimulation).[20] As this stimulation occurs, the release of dopamine in the mesolimbic system inaugurates what Robinson and Berridge call "sensitization," which corresponds to what I have called the *registration* of the object's features and value by the subject. Through sensitization, the object that has just induced dopamine release is recognized and remembered as having done so, through both a physical adaptation of the neurons in the mesolimbic system and a correlative alteration in the perceptual field of the subject. In Robinson and Berridge's words, sensitization is a process that

> transforms the sensory features of ordinary stimuli, or more accurately, the neural and psychological representations of stimuli, so that they become especially salient stimuli, stimuli that "grab the attention," that become especially attractive and wanted, thus eliciting approach and guiding behavior to the goal.[21]

In other words, when an object stimulates the mesolimbic circuits, its status for the subject shifts: no longer an ordinary stimulus, it becomes a *salient* stimulus, a stimulus to which the subject has become sensitized, which means, according to the text just cited, that this is now a stimulus that *grabs* the subject's attention and *elicits* the subject's motion. It is as if the object is highlighted or exaggerated within the visual field of the subject, such that the object takes on—to use a favorite metaphor of Berridge's—a *magnetic* quality for the subject, exerting a pull on the interest as well as movement of the subject. This *pull* on the subject is experienced, by the subject, as *desire* for the object, a desire that is at once internal to the subject—ingrained, as it were, within the nerves of the subject's body—but equally manifest as a real transformation in the perceived object field.

As Robinson and Berridge note, a number of contextual factors "modulate the expression and development of sensitization."[22] In other words, it would be too simple to say that an object has its fixed degree of potency, and that this degree translates into the formation of a certain amount of desire for every subject under every circumstance. For example, it appears that taking a drug in one's home results in a less powerful sensitization (the object is attributed a relatively smaller amount of salience) than taking a drug in unfamiliar settings, and the potency of any given object can be enhanced by its association with other powerfully stimulating objects.[23] Yet the *primary* determinant of whether sensitization will occur, and the degree to which it occurs, is the potency or "reward value" of the object in question and the number of times the subject encounters that object. Thus, "craving"—which, according to the glossary provided by Robinson and Berridge, is not to be understood as a distinct *type* of desire, but rather as the quantitative-maximum form of "wanting"[24]—is to be explained by the incredibly high reward value of addictive objects, on the one hand, and an accumulation of experiences in which the subject is stimulated by and thus sensitized to those objects, on the other. And very often, high reward value and repeat enjoyment go together, not necessarily because the subject consciously seeks out high reward-value objects, but because it is in the nature of highly rewarding objects to produce strong desire for themselves in the subject after only a few experiences of enjoyment. Thus, the answer to the question of addiction is just that "with repeated use drugs gradually become more and more attractive"—through the process of sensitization—"and become increasingly able to control behavior."[25] And it is emphatically not that addicts are chasing pleasure even if the drug no longer brings pleasure, that they have invested the drug with special promise or meaning, or that they are in flight from pain.

What Robinson and Berridge give us, however, is much more than this answer to the question of addiction. Or rather, in answering the question of addiction they give us a theory and figure of the desiring subject in general, one whose wanting is always isomorphic with craving, if usually more moderate in intensity and effect. In a contribution to a volume on the psychology of motivation, Berridge writes that "addiction is a pathological case," both for its extremity and its debilitating social consequences, and yet he takes addiction to exemplify the dynamics of incentive-salience attribution, which he identifies as "crucial to normal reward learning." Attribution is the same process by which we develop desires for "sensory rewards," like "drugs and sex and food," but its purview is much wider than this: "human abstract and cultural and cognitive rewards tap into these same brain systems."[26] And indeed, addiction itself is a potentiality in our relations to all these various rewards and objects, since it is, after all, nothing more than a name for a strong form of desire (and the consequences that unfold in the brain should that desire be satisfied on many repeat occasions), having its conditions in the way the subject desires and the presence, in the world that the subject inhabits, of potently stimulating rewards.

The theory of attribution, and the general figure of desire that it carries, thus constitutes a challenge and innovation, not just in relation to earlier scientific accounts of addictive craving, but also in relation to the broader imagination of desire that was carried in those earlier accounts (and in many non-scientific twentieth-century accounts of addiction). That broader imagination, as I began to describe at the start of this chapter, was one in which desire is understood as a personal and hidden force within each subject, which is supposed to develop in certain normative ways in the course of a life, and whose degree of development within any given subject determines not just the specific tastes but the whole character of that subject. Thus, when addictive craving was reckoned as abnormal desire, and more precisely, as primitive desire, it was understood to be the symptom of a breakdown of character, a regression of mind. I characterized this imagination of desire, which underlay interpretations of craving as primitive desire, as an instance of what Foucault called the *confessional* figure of desire, insofar as it cast desire as something *in* and deep within each subject, and as something deeply *revealing* about the subject whose desire it is, that is, not simply as an accidental aspect of the subject, but as a kind of personal essence and secret, something to be confessed. I now want to consider the theory of attribution, not just as an advance on older theories of addictive desire, but as a move beyond the whole confessional figure of human desire. Comparing the new figure of desire crafted by the attribution theory point-by-point with the confessional figure will help us to grasp precisely what is new in the attribution theory, how it newly imagines us as desiring creatures as it is increasingly accepted as a true account of desire in our day.

In *The History of Sexuality, Volume One*, Foucault theorizes the confessional subject of desire as one whose desire is produced as a "truth [that is] lodged in our most secret nature," and hence capable of being *expressed* in the form of verbal disclosure—"driven from its hiding place in the soul" by means of a "ritual of discourse" in which the subject speaks not only as but also about themselves.[27] This does not mean that such speech is the only manifestation of desire, or that the subject always knows what desire finds expression in their speech, but that desire has the form of a linguistically communicable *meaning* that issues from and can illuminate the inner depths of the speaker—that desire is ultimately revealed by what the subject says that they want, and that in confessing desire, the subject also confesses themselves.

In fact, addiction has long been—and continues to be—an object of confession, in the form of memoirs, in private talk-therapy sessions, in mutual-help associations, and more. And in the twentieth century, speech was indeed a privileged (if surely not exclusive) text from which the unbridled desire for drugs at the heart of addiction could be inferred. Thus, for instance, parents, teachers, and physicians were instructed by anti-drug handbooks in the 1970s and 1980s to listen for traces of hostility, aggression, deceptiveness, and immaturity in the speech of their children, even where physical evidence of chronic drug use could not be found, while talk therapy was a privileged venue for the detection of addiction since, as one practitioner put it, "in therapy, the opportunity to hear someone think out loud about a problem important to him maximizes the opportunity to come to know how he uses or misuses logic, remember clearly or not at all, does or does not exercise good judgment about his own thinking, and whether or not he is able to know his own feelings," all of which is diagnostic of the addict, who tends to "talk glibly, use clichés," and in general to speak in ways that cause one's "head . . . to spin."[28] But most importantly, the *figure* of desire that informed twentieth-century accounts of craving as primitive desire imagined it as formed in and as the psychic character of an individual, and hence as something to be *ex-pressed* from the depths of that person, as a hidden and personally significant secret.

Yet to the extent that incentive-salience attribution is taken to be a truthful account of the subject's desire and its formation, desire is no longer constituted as something to be confessed. It is, of course, still possible to speak about one's desire, but confession will not be the proper form of appearance for desire, and desire will not be a meaning to express. Rather, as we saw, desire is figured—in the theory of attribution and in any of the contemporary media (public, scholarly, and political) that present this theory as the truth of desire—as a *pull* on the subject by the object and as a corresponding *motion* on the part of the subject (a motion that may take the form of a looking, at minimum, and a full approach, at the extreme). Hence, desire becomes something to be *measured* in terms of extent, intensity, or magnitude, not something to be listened to and said. This is not only because desire is, on this theory, mostly "pre-conscious"—desire is, of course, often unconscious for the confessional subject—but because it does not consist in expectations of pleasure or semantically laden wishes, and rather refers to the literal attraction of the subject by the object, the degree to which a given object "elicits approach" for the subject, in Robinson and Berridge's phrase. Hence, the desire of the subject is best captured by "behavioral measures"—records of the subject's actual movement toward the object—and indeed Robinson and Berridge sometimes equate "wanting" with "goal-directed behavior" itself.[29]

Further, what desire reflects, once captured, is no longer the inner constitution or psychic character of the subject. What I want is not a reflection of who I am, because my desire is not the result of a private and continuous developmental history, one in which my yearning for pleasure has been channeled and organized in ways that are socially influenced and yet finally typical of, idiosyncratic to, and more or less enduring for me. Instead, what my desire reflects is the potency of the objects that I have encountered and the record of my encounters with those objects. If I am passionately in pursuit of an object, this tells you, above all, about the reward value of that object and the past and present availability of that object to me, but this telling is not dependent on me, since the truth of my desire is not *my* truth but rather the truth of the *object* to which I have been sensitized—its capacity to recruit and elicit approach from not just me, but any number of me's.

In this way, desire is *de-verbalized* and *de-personalized*, and the subject of this desire is no longer a confessional subject. This subject is the site of its desire, but not quite the source of its desire, and although its desire may be deeply ingrained—inscribed in the neural circuits, and not easily reworked or erased—it does not live in an idealized psychic depth that realizes itself in the phenomenal life of the subject. Rather, that desire has its reality fully within the phenomenal field (as a neurological configuration, on the one hand, and as the attractions of an object world, on the other) and it is thus measurable by tracing the physical contours of that field—or rather, by tracing the way those contours are followed out by the subject's gaze and comportment. Thus, the account of the desiring subject constructed and circulated by the theory of attribution is one that profoundly revises the confessional figure presumed in earlier accounts of craving that cast it as an immature or primitive desire. To the extent that the attribution theory is accepted as true, desire becomes something to be measured in behavioral intensities, not disclosed in rituals of speech; it signifies the power of objects rather than the subject's particular character or personality; and it takes shape as the visible motion of our bodies, not as the telling impulse of a soul, its secret.

In fact, the extent of the attribution theory's acceptance in late-modern American society is wide and daily growing, as it continues to be affirmed and disseminated in scholarly articles, medical textbooks, public-health reports, and popular primers as an explanation for addictive craving. And this development,

I want to suggest, may be read as one way in which desire and the desiring subject are being *de-confessionalized*—constructed anew on a model precisely at odds with the confessional figure of desire—in our time. But crucially, it is not the only way. At this point, I would like to make a turn in this chapter, and broaden our inquiry beyond the domain of contemporary reflections on addiction. Studying the attribution theory in detail has given us the narrative form of de-confessionalization, but this narrative form can explain much more than the significance of this particular theory's rise and dissemination. In fact, I now want to argue that the de-confessionalization of desire as achieved through the rise and dissemination of the theory of attribution can serve as a prism for a number of important changes in the social practices and cultural languages through which desire is observed, evaluated, and constructed in the late-modern United States. It may be that the de-confessionalization of desire is, in fact, an ascendant or at least recurrent phenomenon in our time which is instanced or reflected in, but not original to, the normalization of addiction. It may be a broader trend, like the emergence of post-disciplinary powers traced in the previous chapter, pertaining to the construction and handling of the subject and its life in our time.

In order to make this last point, I now want to take leave of the domain of addiction to consider three other instances of de-confessionalization in contemporary US society: the emergence of cognitive behavior therapy as the dominant form of psychotherapy; the rise of self-tracking as a popular means of self-knowledge and self-exploration; and the ubiquitous use of ratings as metrics to measure the attractiveness or desirability of objects in our day. It is worth emphasizing, at the outset, that I do not see these four developments (including the novel theorization of craving) as identical, or as causally related to one another. Nor do I see them as equally perfect instances of what, in developing a conceptual account of how the desiring subject is reconstituted by recent innovations in addiction science, I have called the process of de-confessionalization. Nonetheless I gather them together because each of these developments represents a historical process, which has occurred in the last half century, wherein a particular construction of the desiring subject on the model of the confessional subject has been displaced along roughly the lines that we saw in the case of addiction science. In other words, each of the developments to be examined shortly is an instance of a historical process that, first, involves a reimagination of the desiring subject, and second, reimagines the desiring subject in a way that is *roughly isomorphic*, or *convergent*, with the process that we studied at length in the case of addiction science, and that is comprehended in its broad outlines by the notion of de-confessionalization. In tracking this rough isomorphism, or convergence, I do not mean to suggest that de-confessionalization is an exhaustive process in our time, one that is potentially occurring everywhere; I do not mean to suggest that the changes enacted by the rethinking of addictive craving are a microcosm of a fully general reconstruction of the desiring subject in our midst. Yet I do mean to argue, as Foucault did with respect to the modern sciences of sexuality, that the reimagination of desire through the science of craving is not entirely unique in its broad outlines, that it can help to illuminate the significance of several other recent changes in our society and culture, and that the acceptance of a de-confessionalized figure of the desiring subject as true, as it is constructed by contemporary theories of craving, is likely abetted and conditioned (although not caused) by the fact that this figure is produced as a truth about us by several influential bodies of knowledge and related practices in our time.

With this set of qualifications and purposes in mind, let us now turn to see how each of the sociocultural developments that I have named enacts the process of de-confessionalization, each in its own way, yet roughly along the lines that I have already outlined. What follows is not meant to be an exhaustive list, but rather a sampling of instances of de-confessionalization occurring in domains or theoretical contexts that are influential for the way many ordinary persons now think about, evaluate, and handle their own desire. Across their differences, the commonalities that we will need to track closely are, to recapitulate, these: the refiguring of desire as a reflection of an object's qualities, rather than an expression of the subject's personality or soul; the realization of desire as manifest behavior and not as obscure meaning; and the use of quantitative measure as the proper form of expression for desire, and no longer verbal self-disclosure.

Cognitive Behavior Therapy

The rise and dissemination of psychoanalysis as theory and practice was one of the key instances for Foucault's thesis that the West was becoming a confessional society, and the Western subject a confessional animal. Indeed, besides Catholic penance, the ritual confession of desire was nowhere more fully realized than in the psychoanalytic clinic, where the free associations of the patient on the couch would be read and interpreted by the analyst for evidence of deep character and psychic formation. Thus, the rise of cognitive behavior therapy (CBT) as the dominant modality of psychotherapeutic practice and its explicit eclipse of the analytic approach—both in theory and practice—over the past half century in the United States may be read as a significant challenge to the confessional figure of desire and the desiring subject. This has been a challenge, moreover, with wide social ramifications. After all, as we saw in the case of addiction, the influence of the analytic framework for desire in the twentieth-century United States went far beyond therapy alone—it was the perspective offered by psychoanalysis and ego psychology that allowed addictive desire to be theorized and treated as primitive desire, and through the prism of the confessional subject. Yet the significance of the rise of CBT exceeds its rejection of psychoanalysis; it consists, as well, in CBT's construction of the desiring subject in a novel form.

If desire was something to be confessed by the subject in the psychoanalyst's clinic, this was because subjective desire was imagined to refract and symptomatize a patient's instinctual history— the way the subject's original instinctual impulses had become restrained, reformed, or channeled by the higher psychic and external social agencies over time.[30] This history, in turn, was taken to comprise the formation of the subject's ego, or "I," in its individuality: the course taken by the drives in the course of early development sets the ground for who one will be. We might take, as a concise formulation of this view, Freud's statement in the *Three Essays on the Theory of Sexuality* that "what we describe as a person's 'character' is built up to a considerable extent from the material of sexual excitations and is composed of instincts that have been fixed since childhood, of constructions achieved by means of sublimation, and of other constructions, employed for effectively holding in check perverse impulses which have been recognized as unutilizable."[31] Here, Freud's point is partly that morality and sexuality are intimately connected, but it is also that what is distinctive about a person, what characterizes them as an individual, is the result of the idiosyncratic fixations and constructions by which their instincts have been organized since childhood. These early fixations and constructions rework the original instincts in ways that are later refracted in the subject's conscious and unconscious desires. Hence, these desires become a kind of text to be read and deciphered in order to arrive at the individuality of the desiring subject, a text produced in the therapist's clinic by being verbally disclosed.

It was precisely a rejection of this way of reading both desire in particular and speech in general that laid the ground for CBT's development. Consider here the reflections of Aaron Beck and Albert Ellis, the two figures generally recognized as the founders of CBT. In a retrospective account of CBT's formation, Beck writes that his search for a new therapeutic approach emerged from his disillusion with "the psychoanalytic unconscious motivational and therapeutic method." In particular, Beck's frustrations in applying the analytic method (he was trained as an analyst) led him to reject the idea that psychopathology can be explained by the developmental history of one's instincts, and he sought to interpret symptoms instead purely on the basis of present and directly observable causes. "Differentiating the cognitive from the psychoanalytic approach," he writes, involved "focusing the treatment on present problems, as opposed to uncovering hidden traumas from the past, and on analyzing accessible rather than unconscious psychological experiences."[32]

At the level of therapy, this entailed a transformation in the evidentiary value and status of a patient's speech. No longer was the patient's disclosure to be read for traces of desire, taken as vehicles of instinct; rather, it would be read for what Beck has called "*idiosyncratic cognitive structures*" or "*schemas*"—the primary material, in his theory, of which the psyche is composed. That is, for Beck, the psyche is not a layered edifice that contains and orders the drives. Rather, it is a kind of lens or grid that filters and interprets the "kaleidoscopic array of stimuli" that arrive to the subject from the world.[33] Schemas, which are learned or internalized continually over time and of which there are many in any individual psyche, are like the "major premises" that attach to the "minor premises" that are environmental stimuli, and everything that one thinks, feels, and otherwise experiences is a "conclusion" of this psychic activity.[34] Thus, psychopathology is not the manifestation of a past instinctual formation; it is, according to Beck, the product of improper schema-application that fully takes place in the present. To continue his metaphor, a pathological symptom is akin to "a recurrent erroneous conclusion" that results from the improper application of an otherwise legitimate schema to an illegitimate occasion, or from the application of a fully illegitimate schema to any number of occasions.[35] Hence, the patient's speech is no longer to be read for evidence of instinct, but rather for the "inaccuracies, misinterpretations, and distortions" in schema-activity that give rise to symptoms such as debilitating fears, anxieties, compulsions, and fantasies, and that speech will be a text from which "one can infer," not character, but "the content of the idiosyncratic schema"—schematic idiosyncrasy takes the place of individuality as the cause and sense of pathology.[36]

Albert Ellis's arrival at CBT proceeded along like lines. Trained in psychoanalysis, Ellis found in his early practice that "the miracle of depth therapy . . . never quite materialized." Even if patients could accept and metabolize his interpretations of their psychic histories, none seemed to achieve lasting emotional relief. Thus, Ellis too began to doubt that pathological symptoms have their roots in the instincts, and located their basis instead in the presence of certain "underlying beliefs" or "axioms" in the minds of patients that distort their experience of reality.[37] He writes that such axioms function as "definitional concepts" that render raw experience intelligible, but in partial and sometimes improperly biased ways. Psychopathology is, again, what results from a disturbing, because illegitimate, rendering of experience by the psyche: patients "*assume*" (albeit unconsciously) a certain premise about their world, "*look* for the 'facts' to prove [the] premise," and then produce (still without knowing) "unvalidated sentences" that register as painful affect ("I am worthless"), obsession ("I must have the object"), and so forth. Ellis writes that "it is these sentences which really *are*, which *constitute* [the patient's] neuroses"—"all human disturbances seem to be of the same definitional nature."[38] Hence, the practice of therapy, in accordance with Ellis's theory, will be much the same as it is for Beck: the therapist reads the patient's speech but also their behavior for their propositional content and traces these back to faulty statements produced in the present by the joining up of psychic schema, or premise, and world.

How, then, is the subject of desire constructed within the theory and practice of CBT, at least in its founding visions? It should be clear that desire loses its capacity to signify the psychic individuality of the patient, both because that individuality is no longer figured as character (and instead as idiosyncratic set of schemas or premises) and because desire is no longer a privileged form of psychic expression. Instead, desire is one of several conclusions or sentences produced, as all psychic phenomena are produced, by the interaction of adopted psychic schemas with the raw material of experience—a production that is thus fully borne and lived out by the subject, but not fully *personal* to that subject, that is, not an *expression* of that subject's core personality but rather the contingent product of a schema that has been adopted by the subject, on the one hand, and the stimulation of the object world, on the other. Thus, we find that the desire of the subject in the CBT clinic is no longer a secret to be confessed and deciphered for meaning, but rather an occasion for the "stereotyped or repetitive patterns of conceptualizing" that may manifest just as well in the forms of behavior, cognition, attention, and more. Desire is, further, here figured as a response of the subject to the impingement of a stimulus or object, as mediated by the schema, and not as an emanation from an inner psyche and soul. And the desire of this subject is, as it were, transposable to other subjects: after all, a major premise or axiom is cognizable by *any* subject, is not tied to any individual subject—hence, my desire is my own in the sense that I have assumed the schema and applied it to the stimulus whose combination gives rise to this desire, but not in the sense that this desire reveals or belongs to me. In these ways, the emergence and dissemination of CBT does not simply push aside psychoanalysis as a theory and practice; it reconstructs the subject presumed and produced by psychoanalysis, giving it a novel, de-confessionalized form.

Self-Tracking

The emergence and dissemination of self-tracking as a popular technique for the production of knowledge about the subject has also occasioned the de-confessionalization of desire in the United States over the past thirty years. It was in the late 1980s that workers in the computer industry began to build and experiment with technologies intended to produce self-knowledge in the form of data; since then, both the equipment and habits of self-knowledge by means of tracking have become ubiquitous in schools, workplaces, and everyday experience as that technology has become fully quotidian—today, over 80 percent of the American population (and over 90 percent of those under fifty) owns a smartphone, and hence has ready access to an instrument for tracking themselves.[39] Indeed, one can now purchase monitors and trackers for physical activity, work productivity, learning outcomes, consumption habits, and more in retail as well as virtual app stores; tracking technologies are installed by default in many workplaces and schoolrooms; and self-tracking has even become the organizing center of cultural subgroups ranging from the techies who "hack" their lives to the so-called "health goths."[40] Although personal health remains the only domain of life in which a large majority of Americans now track themselves daily, self-tracking as a cultural phenomenon is not limited to any particular domain. In her analysis of the English-language media coverage of self-tracking in recent decades, the sociologist Deborah Lupton finds that "by 2012, news articles represented quantified-self practices as growing in popularity and becoming not only an important feature of health promotion but a part of everyday life, as a way of maximizing productivity and happiness as well as health."[41]

To be sure, self-tracking does not obviate alternative means of self-knowing, in the way that CBT claims to have rendered psychoanalysis not just inferior but obsolete. And yet what is significant for my purposes here is how the subject is figured where and when it is the object of self-tracking. To see this, I want to consider the discourse of the Quantified Self community, an online organization with in-person regional chapters that is mostly responsible for elaborating the theoretical framework of self-tracking, and has functioned, according to Lupton, as "the public face" of self-tracking as a cultural movement.[42] In particular, let us examine the point and premise of self-tracking as a mode of "self-knowledge through numbers" as it is elaborated in a 2010 article in the *New York Times Magazine* authored by Gary Wolf, cofounder of Quantified Self and the best-known promoter of this novel practice.

According to Wolf, the development of self-tracking over the past forty years cannot be reduced to the popularization of a marginal pastime. It is, rather, the culmination of a centuries-long historical process. Modernity itself, he argues, is an epoch in which "the fetish for numbers" takes hold of an ever-increasing range of human experience.[43] This fetish first established itself "in science, in business, and in the more reasonable sectors," as quantitative metrics became both the gold standard of evidence and the proper medium of communication in each sphere. From there, the fetish for numbers conquered nearly every other field, until "only one area of human activity appeared to be immune": "personal life." For most of the twentieth century, "the imposition, on oneself or one's family, of a regime of objective record keeping seemed ridiculous." This domain alone remained under the sway of the fetish for language, so that if "a journal was respectable," "a spreadsheet was creepy." In our time, this has changed. Today, "numbers are infiltrating the last redoubts of the personal," as ordinary people now render in numbers their "sleep, exercise, sex, food, mood, location, alertness, productivity, even spiritual well-being."

More than a shift of technology, the move from language to numbers produces a novel figure of the self to be known. "A hundred years ago, a bold researcher fascinated by the riddle of human personality might have grabbed onto new psychoanalytic concepts like repression and the unconscious," and then rendered the human itself in linguistic form: "these ideas were invented by people who loved language" and hence held that "the road to knowledge [about the self] lies through words." This meant that "even as therapeutic concepts of the self spread" beyond the sphere of psychoanalysis "they retained something of the prolix, literary humanism of their inventors." One conceived the self in "literary" terms, that is, as a meaning to be expressed or disclosed in language. This entire vision is what self-tracking displaces. "Trackers are exploring an alternate route. Instead of interrogating their inner worlds through talking and writing, they are using numbers." And against the literary self, "they are constructing a quantified self."

What is the desire of the quantified self? To begin with, it is not a secret: "When we quantify ourselves, there isn't the imperative to see through daily existence into a truth buried at a deeper level." But that does not mean that desire is easily seen. For desire, just like the rest of human interiority, is not an obvious fact or visible in a single instance. Rather, it is something to be observed over time, something indicated much more by what one does and how one responds to certain conditions, rather than by what one may profess or even perform at any given moment. Consider the example of one self-tracker featured on the Quantified Self website, who wanted to "definitively prove my love for my husband and not somebody else" by means of a tracking experiment.[44] Years into her marriage, she knew what she consciously felt, and yet sought proof of her desire in numbers. She began by producing a data set tracking her behavior, retroactively, by converting all her chat messages from her computer into a searchable plain-text database. She then searched, in this data, for what she calls a "sign of love," not by probing what she said for what she meant, but by tracking her patterns of verbal behavior. She considered how often she typed her husband's name, relative to other words; how often and what times of day she wrote to her husband, relative to colleagues and friends; the number of words that were unique to her chat history with her husband; and so forth. Each would signify love, not by surfacing what lay in the tracker's heart, but by revealing intense or otherwise privileged forms of engagement. Desire *is*, in this experiment, a particular pattern of behavior; the task is "to see if there was love *present in my chatting behavior*."[45]

The point here is not that this self-tracker *believes* that love is reducible to behavior. (She may or may not.) It is that the figure of the self constructed by the discourse and practice of self-tracking is one whose interiority is not a psychic depth, but rather habitual patterns of behavior charted over time. In Natasha Dow Schüll's phrase, in the techniques of self-tracking, "bits and moments, accumulating into habits, rhythms, and tendencies, are the 'stuff' of the self," and this is as true of one's desire as it is of one's capacity for productivity, one's attentiveness to one's children, and one's mental health.[46] The premise, and the promise, of self-tracking is that these aspects of our inner worlds will be disclosed, not by what we say, which is always liable to error and distortion, but by what we do, and especially by what we do as it gathers into patterns over time. Thus, where self-disclosure for the sake of self-knowledge takes the form of the tracked record, rather than the first-person narrative or diaristic revelation, the subject is imagined and registered explicitly not as a confessional animal—that literary self is here suspended, if not refused. As we know ourselves by tracking ourselves, we render our desire, once again, in a de-confessionalized form: as a desire that is borne by, but not born within, the subject; as a desire whose truth is acted out rather than hidden within; and as a desire that is therefore capturable by metrics and not only, indeed not well, by the medium of expressive language.

Rating

One of the main features of what many have called our financialized contemporary world is the ubiquitous use of ratings as a measure of value. Today, ratings are produced and consulted as a primary metric for expressing the value of consumer goods, financial products, and commercial experiences, but also of such things as beauty and art, education, intellectual products, and the standing, trustworthiness, and future promise of individual persons. It may seem unintuitive to think of ratings as an expression of *desire*, as well, but consider that the value captured by the value-form of ratings is the capacity of the rated object to attract investors, both now and in the future, and hence can also be understood as the *attractiveness* of the rated object. The rating, in short, reflects past and present desire for what is being rated, as well as the likelihood that the rated object will retain its ability to attract desire in the future—a fact made especially plain, as we will see, in ratings of personal attractiveness.

But let us ask, once again, what figure of subjective desire is capturable in the rating? Revealing here is the ongoing trend among online platforms to replace star-rating systems with a binary system in which the object is rated with a "thumbs-up" or "thumbs-down."[47] Consider, for instance, the widely publicized decision by Netflix to make this change in 2017. "Five stars feels very yesterday now," insisted Todd Yellin, a senior executive at the company.[48] The main problem with the star-system, he explained, was that users tended to employ ratings as a form of self-expression, that is, as a way of indicating the kind of content that they would want to have associated with their identity or personality. Yet the purpose of ratings is to demonstrate the value of new products, meaning their actual capacity to attract the attention and engagement of users. Yellin explained: "We're spending many billions of dollars on the titles we're producing and licensing, and with these big catalogs, that [magnitude] just adds a challenge. Bubbling up the stuff people *actually want to watch* is super important."[49] For ratings to achieve this "bubbling up"—that is, for them to capture the real value and attractiveness of new titles—they cannot be used to show what one wants others to *think* that one wants to watch. "What's more powerful" in this regard, asks Yellin: "you telling me that you would give five stars to the documentary about unrest in the Ukraine; that you'd give three stars to the latest Adam Sandler movie; or that you'd watch the Adam Sandler movie 10 times more frequently?" "What you do versus what you say you like are different things," Yellin concludes, and it is the former that the implementation of the binary system is supposed to help the ratings capture and expose.

Notice that in the course of Yellin's speech, three things become importantly confused, substituting for one another. First, ratings are intended to convey a user's *desire*, what they "want to watch"; but second, this desire is construed as equivalent with what they *do* watch, rather than what they say or think about themselves; and third, what their desire discloses is the probability of their watching, in the future, what they are watching now. Thus, desire is construed, by the Netflix rating, as equivalent with behavior and actual investment of attention, which is why the effectiveness of the rating system can be checked by comparison to measures of past activity: according to Yellin, one reason for the company's decision to shift to the binary system was that its results better aligned with what Netflix could already glean from analyzing users' browsing histories. And this desire is employed as a measure, not of who the audience is or what they want as a collective subjectivity, but rather what the value of the object is—its capacity to attract and hold the attention of viewers.

Obviously, a Netflix rating is not the same thing as a credit rating, a college rating, or a swipe across the Tinder screen. But in each case, the rating measures, and in doing so *figures*, our desire as a response to an attractive object much more than an expression of personality. Desire is, in other words, a reflection of the *desirability* of the object, not something formed within and specific to me. The Tinder rating is an especially good example of this. Generally, users cannot view their own personal ratings, but the company does assign one to each user in order to enable pairings among similarly "desirable" individuals. Here is how the system works, as explained by a journalist: "You rose in the ranks based on how many people swiped right [on] ('liked') you, but that was weighted based on who the swiper was. The more right swipes that person had, the more their right swipe on you meant for *your* score. Tinder would then serve people with similar scores to each other more often, assuming that people whom the crowd had similar opinions of would be in approximately the same tier of what they called 'desirability.'"[50] Note that here again, what one desires is registered by what one does—one's "opinion" of desirability is not spoken but "swiped"—and what the rating reveals is the desirability of the rated object, not the identity of the swipers, who meld into the figure of a "crowd." What one wants is not a secret and it is not personal; it is evident in one's behavior and incited by the valuable object.

As ratings become an ever-more ubiquitous form of expression for desire and desirability in our culture, these latter lose their indexical relation to personalities, and become exchangeable across *any* subject that encounters the rated object. Indeed, as we have seen, the desire registered by a rating is *predictive* of the desire of another subject, whoever they are, since my desire is nothing more than how this object engages me or leads me to act: the desire that I experience is the desire of a crowd; it is impersonal and on the surface, rather than a sign of what moves me as a result of my constitution or my history. This figure of desire becomes legible wherever ratings take hold as a major practice. Consider one final example: the philosopher Michel Feher's recent argument that ratings might become a prominent form of political agency in this century. Taking inspiration from the divestment campaign waged against the Keystone Pipeline, Feher suggests that "in a speculative age," battles over political power must aim at "altering the conditions of accreditation" much more than the conditions of wage-labor.[51] This means that we must exercise a "rated agency," that is, our capacity "to speculate with other like-minded investees on what assets should be recognized as appreciable and thus on who deserves to be called creditworthy," and to do this, tangibly, through "the collection of information and the publication of 'opinions' on the risks of an investment."[52] Feher is compelling, in my view, but notice what happens to the political tract in this exercise of agency: we give voice to our desire to divest from organizations and projects that are exploitative or that work against environmental sustainability, but this desire is voiced as a measure of the *undesirability* (the non-appreciability or low creditworthiness) of the object, rather than as an expression of who we are as a people. The subject of this desire is a faceless subject, one that does not confess its desire but seeks to publish it, as a reflection of what it rates much more than who is rating. The desire of the rating subject thus converges with that of the addicted subject, the therapeutic subject, and the self-tracking subject in its impersonality, its responsiveness to the object, and its capacity to be observed and registered in numerical metrics. It is, yet again, an instance of the de-confessionalization of the desiring subject, one of several, I hope to have shown, that has unfolded over the past four decades in US society.

For Foucault, the project of theorizing the confessional figure of desire and the desiring subject served two crucial purposes. First, it enabled him to reveal the dual significance, or achievement, of the modern sciences of sex. Not only did they offer new accounts of sexual life in particular; they produced a new understanding of desire and the desiring subject in general. And second, the notion of a confessional figure of desire allowed Foucault to cast the rise of the modern sexual sciences as one part of a larger cultural transformation in the eighteenth- and nineteenth-century West. This transformation, not unified and yet widespread, was the appearance in those centuries of an increasing number of diverse bodies of knowledge that construed desire as a hidden secret of each person to be confessed and, accordingly, of social occasions for the confession of personal desire. Foucault went so far as to speak of a transformation of the West, in the eighteenth and nineteenth centuries, into a "singularly confessing society," that is, a society in which the Catholic imperative established in the seventeenth century—"Not only will you confess to acts contravening the law, but you will seek to transform your desire, your every desire, into discourse"[53]—had become a generalized imperative, one imposed upon individuals or tacitly expected in venues such as "justice, medicine, education, family relationships," and more.[54] Far from being a special theory of the modern sexual sciences, the figure of desire as something confessed, and of the desiring subject as a potential confessant, became a commonplace in modern Western societies, and even, Foucault suggests, desire's most familiar and dominant form.[55]

Thus the confessional figure of desire was for Foucault not just a device for interpreting the modern sexual sciences, but also part of a historical narrative concerning the construction of desire most typical of the modern West. We need not accept the provocatively totalizing rhetoric of his narrative in order to acknowledge its partial and illuminating truth. One sign of its truth is the fact that the confessional figure of desire readily captures the four figures of desire that each of the developments examined in this chapter cast as hegemonic in the nineteenth and twentieth centuries in the United States, and that each seeks to overturn and displace. I cite the cultural-historical dimension of Foucault's theorization of the confessional figure of desire here because recalling it allows us to see a larger possible significance in the de-confessionalizations of desire that we have traced. If the confessional figure of desire was not just one local imagination, but *a* or even *the* commonplace construction of desire in modern Western societies, then perhaps the fact that desire is now being de-confessionalized in a diverse range of domains in late-modern US society is something more than an interesting recurrence. Perhaps it indicates a shift, as well, in what counts as a conventional construction of desire in our society, a shift reflected in and furthered by the normalization of addictive craving, the rise of cognitive behavior therapy, the popularization of self-tracking, and the dissemination of ratings, but that goes beyond any one of them. Let me end this chapter with this more speculative claim about the construction of desire in late-modern America, extending, as it were, Foucault's story about desire in the modern West.

Perhaps in late-modern American society, confession is less and less a means for giving expression to our desire, and desire itself is less and less conceived as the sort of thing that subjects can or ought to confess. This would explain at least one curious development now occurring in the clinics of psychoanalysis, which have not disappeared but rather still exist on the margins of American society as places where confessing one's desire remains, or is supposed to remain, a crucial practice. The prominent psychoanalyst Christopher Bollas has written in a recent book that an odd new type of patient has been "on the rise" in Europe and the United States since the "third quarter of the [twentieth] century." This is a type of patient that Bollas used to diagnose in earlier decades as suffering from what he, drawing on the work of the psychoanalyst Joyce McDougall, called "normopathy," a condition that now seems extremely common, thus perhaps less an individual affliction than a state proper to and induced by the present epoch. The normopath is characterized by a variety of symptoms, such as an obsession with material objects, a tendency to accumulate facts and data, and a muted response to traumatic events, but the "fundamental characteristic" of this figure is "a lack of interest in subjective life" that constitutes a kind of immunity to interpretive analysis.[56] One exemplary patient responds, to Bollas's interpretation of her persistent desire to become indispensable to significant others: "You got it. . . . That's brilliant—thanks so much," as if the psychoanalyst were less a diver of subjective depths than "a good auto mechanic or computer expert."[57] There is no confession to be anticipated, let alone forced, in this scene—not because the subject is unwilling to confess but because the subject seems to have nothing to confess, and the admission of her desire induces no effect, revealing nothing more than a fact of her existence, and surely not signifying a secret that only desire might express. Indeed, McDougall first theorized the normopathic patient in order to describe a sort of person "becoming ever more frequent in today's practice." Tellingly, her other name for this sort of person was "the anti-analysand."[58]

What if we were to take the reports of Bollas and McDougall as true? Perhaps we might hazard this guess, as a partial explanation: It may be that if desire is increasingly difficult to confess, even in a domain that continues to construct desire on the model of the confessional subject, this is not just because, as Bollas himself suggests, people are led in an overwhelming and unfathomably distressing world to turn away from introspection, to lose interest in internal phenomena, to "turn away from subjectivity."[59] Perhaps it is rather that the patients who enter the psychoanalyst's clinic are increasingly ones who have learned to see and interpret their inner desires in ways incompatible with the confessional construction that they encounter in the psychoanalyst's clinic. Perhaps what allowed clinical confession to work so well in the last century, what lent it therapeutic efficacy as well as prestige, was not simply the force of the analyst's discourse alone, but the preparation of patients for internalizing and making use of that discourse as a means of self-understanding and self-interpretation by a whole culture, a singularly or at least ubiquitously confessing society, in which a wide range of knowledges, practices, and everyday precepts about human experience impressed upon those patients, prior to their becoming patients, that desire is a thing that lies latent in each of us, that it is our secret and personal meaning, and that in order to be handled and assessed, desire has to be laid bare in language—it is something to be, and that must be, confessed. Perhaps what Bollas is observing in the clinic—not a resistance, but an incapacity to confess—reflects the changed culture of a *late*-modern society, which no longer prepares or expects us to confess our desires, or to have a kind of desire that is amenable to being confessed. Perhaps what he is seeing reflects a new social age, with a new set of conventions, formed by the emergence of a variety of new knowledges and social practices that presume and explicitly claim that desire is precisely not something that reveals us, not a hidden secret, and not something to be confessed. Perhaps the de-confessionalization of desire is more than the common meaning of the developments studied in this chapter, but a trend, and even an ascendant framework for figuring our desire, and figuring ourselves as subjects of desire, in the late-modern United States. Such is the fullest context, I propose, for understanding the reimagination of craving as a norm of desire in our recent history, that is, for developing the whole of its possible sense and significance.

FOUR

Reframing the Self
Addiction and Wellness

This chapter revisits and rethinks a historical development that is separable from, yet deeply linked with, the normalization of addiction, namely, what scholars have called the "expansion" of addiction discourse in the United States over the last forty years.[1] From the days of the Temperance Movement through most of the twentieth century, reference to addiction in the United States was bound by what scholars call its "restrictive meaning," which reserves the term only for cases of compulsive substance use involving severe tolerance and withdrawal.[2] Yet in the past half century, addiction discourse has become both promiscuous and ubiquitous. Not only are substance addictions now diagnosable in the absence of any specific physiological markers, so too are intense involvements with sex, technology, work, shopping, eating, gaming, and more both widely self-described and clinically identified as addictions. Medical researchers have begun investigating such things as carrot and tanning addictions, while the prevalence of familiar addictions only continues to increase.[3] "Addiction has crept into the crevices of our culture," observe two leading social theorists of addiction: "we hear it everywhere"; it has assumed "a prominent place in our lexicon."[4]

It is not hard to see how the expansion of addiction discourse is linked to the normalization of addiction. It is linked in at least three ways. First, the expansion of addiction discourse refers, in part, to a sheer increase in volume of texts, talk, and public representations of addiction. To the extent that this growth has occurred at a time when scientific, medical, and political constructions that normalize addiction have become more common and mainstream, the expansion of addiction discourse can be seen, at least in part, as a dissemination in American society of normalizing constructions of addiction. Second, the expansion of addiction discourse refers to an increase in the number of addictions that are now recognized in public media, medicine, and scholarship. In general, new addictions are established by analogizing hitherto disparate conditions to drug and alcohol addictions. As Mark Griffiths writes in the article that launched the study and treatment of technological addictions, "the way of determining whether technological addictions are addictive in a non-metaphorical sense is to compare them against clinical criteria for other established [i.e., substance] addictions."[5] Thus, to the extent that, as we have seen, normalizing constructions of addiction have become central to addiction science and diagnostic practice, the articulation of new types of addiction brings the knowledge that addiction is normal to new life spheres. And finally, the growth of talk about addiction and the increasing number of addictions to which we are liable themselves lend credence to the idea that addiction is a normal part of human existence. If we are addicted so often and in so many ways, so much the more plausible is it to think that we are addictive creatures by nature. As a recent scholarly review of prevalence estimates for the various addictions concludes: "a high prevalence of some type of addiction among a significant minority of the population might suggest that addiction is a natural state of affairs as a human being."[6] In short, the expansion of addiction discourse is, in part, an expansion precisely of normalizing constructions of addiction; and further, it is itself evidence of addiction's normalcy.

If the ways in which the expansion of addiction discourse contributes to the normalization of addiction are clear, less obvious is what motivates this development in the first place. Why have so many addictions, and new types of addiction, been claimed and identified, in so many different domains of experience, in recent decades? Many other scholars have posed this question, and their answers have tended to interpret the expansion of addiction discourse in the way that Marx read the clamor of religion: as the lament of an oppressed creature who feels impotent but cannot properly diagnose this feeling. The critic Stanton Peele, for instance, writes that the sharp growth of the addiction treatment industry and of the general cultural consciousness of addiction "expresses the loss of control that we have developed as a society" in an age of elite-run politics, splintered communities, decline of tradition, and so forth.[7] Anthony Giddens and Eve Kosofsky Sedgwick make a similar analysis at the individual level: the "epidemic of addiction attribution," in their accounts, registers a widening sense of personal failure to realize the ideals of liberal autonomy so valorized in the West.[8] Others interpret our expanding addiction discourse as a reflection of life under a new phase of capitalism in which production is not just indifferent to real human need but directly aimed at the most insatiable consumer appetites.[9]

But why should *addiction* be the means of expression for felt impotence in our day? Why should our failures and dispossessions appear to us as so many addictions, rather than as states of madness, alienation, subjection, exploitation, or even sheer decadence? After all, as we will see, in our time addiction is not simply a name for lost control or dispossession; rather, it signifies a more complex state in which one's level of engagement with a particular object or activity is sustained at unusually high levels by an array of inner and outer influences that do not vitiate, but overpower, one's conscious wishes and intention. Moreover, many of the most prominent contemporary scholarly and popular accounts of addiction figure the subject and self in a way that goes against the idea that we are ever simply *in* or *out* of control. Rather, if we are liable to addiction, this is because there is never a directly causal relation between subjective intention and conduct, although that relation is not for that unreal: we are, in a sense to be developed below, understood in such accounts of addiction as always the *agents* but never the *authors* of how we live and what we do. Addiction will turn out to be the name for the most severe and debilitating form that the ever-present gap between the subject's own purposes and its experience can take. Hence, an expanding addiction discourse represents the widening circulation, not quite of a condemnation of ourselves as failing to master our existence, but of this particular way of figuring the human and its ills, one that expresses pain and regret, to be sure, but also a sense that a failure of self-mastery is at some level normal. How do we understand the phenomenon, recast in this way? How do we account for the expansion of addiction discourse once we see that what is expanding in our time is, in large part, a recognition *both* of the fact that addiction is everywhere among us and that the root of addiction is normal?

In answering this question, I will not provide a strictly causal account of the expansion of addiction discourse. Rather, as in previous chapters, I will theorize a broader cultural development in late-modern American society that is reflected in, supportive of, and furthered by the expansion of addiction discourse. This broader development is what I will call the spread of a novel mode of self-relation, or what Foucault calls a modality of "the relationship of self with self," over the last forty years. For Foucault, this term was meant to facilitate recognition and study of the fact that how we experience ourselves—how we see our own bodies, minds, and capacities, and how we think we can act on these—is always socially mediated, always dependent on social frameworks. These frameworks arrive to us, he argued, in the form of texts, theories, and social practices. In *The Hermeneutics of the Subject*, Foucault describes the components of a social framework for the self, or a mode of self-relation, in the following way, taking the Roman mode of *epimeleia heautou* as an exemplary case. First, a mode of self-relation defines "an attitude towards the self, others, and the world," or a "general standpoint" on what self, others, and world are. Second, it defines "a certain form of attention, of looking" at oneself, a way of analyzing and assessing the different parts of the self. And third, it defines a set of possible "actions exercised on the self by the self, actions by which one takes responsibility for oneself, and by which one changes, purifies, transforms, and transfigures oneself."[10] In short, a mode of self-relation defines what we can see when we look at ourselves, or reflect on ourselves, and how we relate to ourselves in action, how we attempt and succeed in changing our own minds and bodies. Self-experience is not immediate or transparent but coordinated by a social framework: "within [a given] relationship of self to self the formation of a certain type of experience becomes possible."[11]

Of course, there may be several modes of self-relation available within any given society. One may well be given a framework for seeing and acting on oneself by one's religious practice and community that differs from the framework offered by one's doctor or psychiatrist. But sometimes there are modes of self-relation that travel especially widely within a society, and that are accepted by a broad swath of the population, both conceptually and actively, and that thus may be counted as prominent or prevalent modes of self-relation in the context of a whole society. Often, such prominent modes of self-relation gain prominence by being codified and circulated in what Foucault calls a "helpful discourse," a body of texts and speech that provides clear lessons, techniques, and easily communicable metaphors intended to help any person preserve or enhance themselves—their bodily or mental health, their spiritual quality, and their overall sense of well-being.[12] A helpful discourse, especially if it is non-denominational or otherwise non-exclusive in its projected audience and terminology, might carry a mode of self-relation especially widely, and render it, if not a dominant mode, then a more or less general framework for self-experience in the society where the helpful discourse circulates.

In this chapter, I argue that the recent expansion of addiction discourse in the United States has been enabled by, and itself furthers, the rise to prominence of a certain mode of self-relation in our time. Although no single discourse fully captures this relation, I will suggest that it has been most clearly articulated and widely carried by the contemporary helpful discourse and associated health practices of *wellness*, whose emergence and popularization in American society is exactly contemporaneous with the expansion of addiction discourse. My argument is not that addiction discourse is a subset or effect of wellness, but that the mode of self-relation theorized and actively formed by wellness figures the self as a creature for whom addiction is an immanent and normal liability. As we will see, the theory and practice of wellness teaches the self to take itself as a site where a diverse array of forces give shape to an existence that we bear and live out, but do not invent or fully determine, and where our own conscious agency is not a privileged blueprint for our lives, but rather one force contending to shape the self among many. As wellness has become an increasingly available and actively accepted framework for the self in contemporary American society—now circulating in countless books and magazines, government pamphlets, workplace programs, campus centers, health clinics, wellness retreats, and quotidian practices—so too has addiction, a condition that is now increasingly understood exactly as an overpowering of one's conscious intention by the other forces shaping one's existence, become more legible and present as a possible threat in human experience. This growing legibility and presence finds expression, I suggest, in the recent and continuing expansion of addiction discourse in the United States.

This chapter proceeds in two stages. First, it considers the historical development of the helpful discourse of wellness in this country, focusing on how the self is figured as an object of perception and cultivation in the foundational texts of the wellness movement. Second, it turns to the conceptual generalization and proliferation of addiction discourse starting in the late 1970s—precisely the moment when wellness, as discourse and practice, begins to disseminate throughout the country—and explores the relation of these two phenomena to one another. As we will see, the precise form that addiction increasingly takes in the expanding discourse of the past half century (i.e., very often a normalized form, as indicated by the sample of influential texts on addiction that this chapter will study) is one that is made intelligible and persistently threatening by the kind of self that wellness promulgates: addiction is not the only malady that the subject of wellness may suffer, but it is an illness made in the image of that subject's mode of suffering. The chapter concludes by reflecting on the question that has led so many social theorists to study the expansion of addiction discourse in recent years—namely, what constraints this expansion imposes on self-interpretation and self-understanding in late-modern Western societies—affirming the value of this question yet finding that the analysis of this chapter pushes us to answer it along new lines.

The broad historical outlines of the development of wellness in late twentieth-century American culture are well known.[13] The term *wellness* first assumed its contemporary meaning in a 1957 academic article by the US public health official Halbert Dunn, but it was little known until the mid-1970s, when several readers of Dunn's later mass-market publications founded what they called "wellness centers," which offered seminars as well as intensive programs for participants who wished not just to eliminate illness, but to cultivate a broader modality of well-being and health. By the late 1970s, the original centers had begun to attract the attention of journalists and health experts, whose coverage of the centers' activity aided the proselytizing efforts of wellness teachers and participants themselves in circulating the ideas and practices of wellness across US society at large. In 1979, a *60 Minutes* program on the burgeoning wellness movement opened with the remark that wellness is "a word that you don't hear every day"; this was no longer true a decade later, by which time the ideals and practices of wellness centers had spilled out into more general venues: popular journals and magazines, corporate health initiatives, medical research programs and conferences, campus resource centers, and more. Wellness also soon became the organizing rubric for the many new health-enhancing practices popularized in the late twentieth century, from jogging and amateur weightlifting to meditation, postural yoga, Pilates, light therapy, and the use of dietary supplements. Thus, although dictionary experts scorned the novel sense of wellness as improper usage throughout the 1980s, by the next decade their battle was lost, and today the late twentieth-century meaning of wellness is at home in every major English-language dictionary, from *Oxford* to *American Heritage*.[14]

What was this novel, and once scandalous, sense of wellness? To see this, we turn to the work of two figures, each of whom is known as the "father of the wellness movement." The first is Halbert Dunn, who laid the basis for the contemporary meaning of wellness in three medical-journal articles published in the late 1950s. Then chief of a major division within the US Public Health Service, Dunn had grown frustrated with what he called the "negative" approach to health promotion that prevailed at the time. In most government strategy, but also in the culture at large, health seemed to mean nothing more than the "absence of illness," and Dunn saw this notion as unsuited to an age in which "neurotic and functional illnesses," and not spectacular diseases and death, were the main threats to well-being.[15] Thus, Dunn sought to invest in the unfamiliar term *wellness* a new way of seeing health, one that was somewhat amorphous at the start but that would be defined by at least three features. First, wellness would signify not an opposite of illness, but rather "a graduated scale" running from worst to best levels of health. Second, wellness would, at its highest levels, signify the ambitious ideal of "performance at full potential in accordance with the individual's age and makeup." Third, wellness would name not just the *ideal* of "high-level wellness," but also and more crucially the orientation and effort toward it: wellness, Dunn wrote, is "*a direction* in progress toward an ever-higher potential of functioning."[16]

For Dunn, wellness was first and foremost a way of framing *public* health. His task was not quite to change individual consciousness but to enable health officials to identify the "points of attack for raising the levels of wellness" in a population.[17] But how could this be done? How, exactly, could "medicine and public health" really "undertake a multiple and thoroughgoing exploration of the factors responsible for good health," construed as wellness?[18] To do this, Dunn insisted, health knowledge would need to be grounded in a more basic understanding of what the human is and how its life and being are affected. Thus, he elaborated, in a series of early articles and then later in a book-length study titled *High-Level Wellness*, what he took to be "the nature of man," which would serve as "the basis for high-level wellness as a useful concept."[19]

"Man," Dunn insisted on many occasions, "is an organization of energy." The theory and practice of wellness must reflect this primary fact: "any concept of wellness must be dynamic," in a sense to be examined shortly, since "energy is dynamic, and the body is made of energy."[20] In Dunn's view, everything that composes the body—and here the body will stand in for the whole of the self, which Dunn saw as integrated rather than split between soma and soul—is a type of energy. The basic chemical substances that compose the body are, for instance, "energy bound into matter," while the various bodily systems—circulatory, endocrine, lymphatic—represent "energy bound into form." These substances and systems are traversed, moreover, by what Dunn calls "communication energy," such as the electrical impulses carried by nerves. Further, the body as a unit is figured in Dunn's theory as a site for the exchange of energy with the world: everything that the body produces and does is an expression of "expendable energy," while all that the body takes in becomes "stored energy," a reserve for later expression.

Dunn recognizes that his view is rather opaque if taken as a theory of human ontology in itself. But his interest is slightly different: "Even though energy may be a mystery to us," we know that "it has some very definite laws," and this law-governed status of energy is the basis for a theory and practice of wellness. For all energy is governed by the laws of the *fields* within which it flows: think, Dunn suggests, of the conduction and flow of particles within "magnetic fields" and "electrical fields." An "energy field," for Dunn, is "a space traversed by lines of force" that act on whatever enters the field—channeling it, animating it, setting its course and direction. The human, figured as energy, can thus be seen as conducted by a variety of energy fields. These include the magnetic fields of the globe, but also, and more figuratively, the natural environment, as well as "social energy fields" and "personality energy fields."[21] The social field, like any other, channels energy inputs toward some persons and away from others, and it conducts individual expressions of energy toward particular ends and occupations, by means of religious, cultural, economic, and political modes of organization. Personality fields, meanwhile, emanate from each individual or from groups, and they direct the flow of intersubjective exchange: that is, of mood, speech, attachment, interest, and the like.

In short, the key lesson of this metaphysics for the work of wellness is this: "The guidelines . . . of energy fields set the course for the growth and progress of the individual and for the welfare of society."[22] If human being is energy, and all energy is conducted by the various fields within which it exists, then the way of raising levels of wellness is to identify and modify the social, natural, and interpersonal *contexts* within which individuals live: "If mankind is to be well, he must have an environment which is conducive to wellness."[23] So, for instance, at the personal scale, one might rearrange one's work space or ameliorate one's family relations in order to cultivate one's wellness; or, at the level of public health, one might introduce universal education in order to draw out the hidden capacities of all youth, ensure widespread occupational opportunities to fully realize what workers can offer, or clear up congestion in urban spaces to relieve the stress that such conditions impose on those who inhabit them. For Dunn, such an approach to public health was not utopian but built on existing, if marginal, views, such as that expressed in a recent task-force report commissioned by the White House, which argued:

> The areas of social action to promote health include any conditions in the external environment that may impose some stress, such as availability and quality of food, housing, working conditions, opportunity to earn a living, to have an education, and to obtain medical care . . . [as well as] those areas which influence the knowledge and attitudes of an individual, thereby affecting his ability to maintain a healthful internal environment—nutritional, emotional, or psychological.[24]

"Effects of misused and misdirected energy are the cause of psychosomatic illness," Dunn wrote; hence, establishing environmental conditions that give good use and direction to human energies would become, for Dunn, the heart of public health's labors, once oriented to and by wellness.[25]

Dunn's writings would become foundational for the broader movement to come, and yet—perhaps because of their strange metaphysical cast—only with what the historian James Miller calls the "missionary work" of Donald Ardell, our second father figure, would wellness become established throughout popular culture.[26] Ardell's work in wellness began during his time as a journalist, in the late 1970s, when he published a series of articles on the new wellness centers, introducing figures such as John Travis (whose Wellness Resource Center would be featured in the 1979 *60 Minutes* program) and their teachings to a broad public. These articles won him a book contract to cover the burgeoning wellness phenomenon as a whole, which resulted in his 1977 bestseller *High-Level Wellness*, both an explicit homage to Dunn and an attempt to translate Dunn's views into a more accessible program, one that would be compatible with the work of the new wellness centers and with what individuals could be expected to do to promote wellness in the context of their daily lives, at home.[27] It was here that wellness would become a framework within which one observes and acts on oneself, much more than a framework for policy.

Ardell affirmed the broad strokes of Dunn's theory, carrying forward, for instance, the concept of wellness as "so much more than the absence of illness," as involving a "continuum," and as culminating in "a state wherein you actually glow with well-being"— "alive clear to the tips of your fingers," with "energy to burn," and "tingl[ing] with vitality."[28] Ardell also affirmed Dunn's view that wellness is to be cultivated not through the heroic interventions of doctors in critical cases but through the establishment of life contexts conducive to the flourishing of individual capacities. Yet Ardell rejected Dunn's peculiar notion of energy fields, and identified *lifestyle* and *environment* as the contexts that fundamentally shape one's existence, and hence as the primary targets for the work of wellness promotion: "attention to lifestyle and environment offers the most rewarding paths to improved levels of health."[29] Further, Ardell took wellness primarily as an ethic of *individual* action rather than as a theory of public health: "The ethic of active self-responsibility for your well-being is the foundation of a wellness philosophy."[30] For Ardell, wellness is not a practice of government—or if it is, it is a "government of you," by you.[31]

However, this is not an injunction for each individual to bootstrap themselves into high-level wellness. "I do not believe there is a single *cause* of wellness," writes Ardell, "or any one thing you can do to get into it."[32] Ardell acknowledges that there are considerable "social obstacles to a wellness lifestyle," and he devotes a quarter of his book to enumerating cultural and political reforms that could clear at least some of these obstacles away.[33] Nor does Ardell think that anyone's actions are directly effective in determining one's health and life outcomes more generally. Hence it is both possible and desirable "to be 'well' in the midst of illness and dying."[34] In fact, wellness is not really an injunction at all; rather, it is "an attitude, or a context in which to perceive your life"—a way of relating to one's body and way of being.[35] "Think of wellness as a game," Ardell suggests, that you "choose or agree to participate

[in]." It has its "rules, penalties, and rewards, spectators, players, goals," and so forth; it is a framework within which to figure one's self as the site of a possible wellness and to orient one's efforts to promote that wellness of the self.[36]

So the rules that Ardell provides in *High-Level Wellness* are not strict orders, but rather exemplary "principles" gathered under each of five dimensions of wellness. The first dimension is self-responsibility—the ethos of active participation in the wellness game from the start—and the rest fall into two categories: lifestyle and environment.[37] Lifestyle names the contexts that shape one's existence which are composed of one's own habits and ongoing activities. Lifestyle comprises three dimensions of wellness: nutrition, stress management, and physical fitness. In each case, the practice of wellness consists not in directly raising one's levels of physical and emotional health, but rather in cultivating a kind of milieu of one's own activity that is conducive to bodily flourishing and relatively inhospitable to disease. Thus, the task of nutrition is to eat in such a way that one will "nourish the environment of your body's cells" and thereby "better your chances to feel, think, and be well."[38] Likewise, one does not aim at directly reducing the body's stress responses, but rather at "constructing an environment suited for and conducive to . . . stress management," which means not only actively making time and space for stress-relief practices in one's life, but maintaining a repertoire of learned techniques or resources for such relief: yoga, hypnosis, meditation, hot baths and saunas, and more. And again, with fitness, there is no ideal physique or heart rate to achieve, but rather the goal of "an individualized fitness regime" that in general elevates the body's "conditioning."[39] Hence what Ardell calls "lifestyle reform" could be described as tending to one's own patterns of activity as if these were the soil in which the body must grow: eating well, managing stress, and pursuing fitness, one acts on oneself intently yet indirectly, by cultivating the medium of one's daily habits, regimens, and activities.

Environment is the fifth dimension, on its own, but it has "three aspects—the physical, the social, and the personal." It refers to those shaping conditions of an individual's life that are founded and maintained entirely outside one's own self, and which are hence less responsive to reform than the dimensions of lifestyle. Each aspect of the environment comprises the forces that "act upon the individual and enhance or limit health and well-being"; environments are "spaces" made up of "all the stimuli or forces acting upon a person at any point in time."[40] The task here is to remove or avoid, to the extent that one can, the negative or draining stimuli and forces in one's environment. For "a positive environment will help you stay healthy and move toward high-level wellness, whereas a negative environment will block your growth toward well-being and all manner of positive expression." Here Ardell is very much in line with Dunn, and he prescribes the following procedure: first, "increase your sensitivity to all the stimuli that touch upon your senses at any point in time"—that is, recognize "the environments, or spaces, [that] affect all aspects of your life"—and then arrange "those aspects of your spaces which you can control."[41]

Unfortunately, "there are severe limits to what most of us can do to change the physical and social aspects of our larger environments." But "it is both easy and enjoyable to design the personal component of your environment"—the spaces of daily life, like one's home, workplace, leisure activities, and relationships. To the extent that one can, Ardell recommends moving away from toxic physical and social environments—he is wary of big cities—and engaging in things like letter-writing campaigns to eliminate pollution, to open up bikeways, to preserve beautiful landscapes, and so forth. Then, one should focus one's efforts on the personal sphere: here, "space-shaping techniques" might include altering one's commute so as to encounter less street noise on the way to work, arranging one's desk area in a clutter-free and more ergonomic fashion, listening to classical music on one's headphones so as to drown out noxious distractions, and eliminating relationships that disturb one's emotional health. With environment, the task is akin to lifestyle reform in that one alters oneself by way of acting on a milieu, but now the conditions are more tangible, instituted out there and not, as it were, consisting in me, in here.

Wellness, then, is not just a "culture," "industry," "ideology," or "secular morality"[42]; it is also an ethos, or a mode of self-government—a framework in which to perceive and act on

oneself—that has been disseminated both by active proselytiza-
tion and through the numerous practices that it organizes, and
that has become a quotidian feature of the contemporary cultural
landscape in the United States. It is a game, in Ardell's metaphor,
that one plays with oneself, in which one figures the self as the
bearer of a life experience that one does not directly determine,
and that is instead powerfully shaped by the forces exerted by (or
making up) the conditions in which the individual and its life are
embedded. These forces are interpersonal, biological, and natural,
but also cultural, social, and political, and they conduct the life
of the self—what it does, how it feels, its survival—in the sense
that they channel that life, give it shape, direction, and form. Of
course, the self is not a passive observer of this conducting; what
wellness gives the self is a way of intervening in the formation
of its life. But that intervention is never direct, always mediated,
and will take a very specific form within the rules of wellness: one
acts on oneself not by taking oneself in hand, but by contending
with the forces that conduct one's life, through lifestyle reform or
environmental remediation.

This is what we are doing when we follow the precepts of all
the contemporary venues explicitly devoted to wellness: wellness magazines and pamphlets, corporate wellness initiatives,
high school and college wellness programs, as well as the many
wellness centers still in business throughout the nation. But it is
also what we are doing when we engage in the kinds of practices
and regimens that Ardell and other wellness teachers prescribe,
but outside the explicit frame of wellness. Consider that jogging,
amateur weightlifting and other fitness-club activities, postural
yoga, Pilates, tai chi, deep breathing exercises, meditation, use
of dietary supplements and elimination of processed foods, and
even such things as light therapy—all these are practices that proliferated throughout US culture in exactly the same period that
wellness has developed, and that allow us to act on ourselves in
the implicit or explicit framework of wellness today.[43] One might
add to this list the sharp and ongoing increase in popular use of
psychopharmaceuticals—amphetamines, anxiolytics, and other
means of mental calibration—since the 1970s, alongside a huge
growth, as well, in the use of illicit drugs.[44] If we understand well-

ness not just as a specific philosophy or a set of sanctioned principles, but as a broader way of figuring, relating to, and cultivating the self as a pliant body conducted by the various conditions (natural, biochemical, cognitive, interpersonal, social, cultural, economic) in which it is embedded, then we can see the ambit of wellness in contemporary culture as much wider than it might first seem. Wellness, then, becomes the name for a mode of self-relation—a way of looking at the self, a way of acting on the self, a repertoire of practices for forming and transforming the self— that frames a great deal of subjective experience in the contemporary United States, one in which we appear as the kind of creature for whom, as we now turn to see, addiction is an increasingly worrisome and imminent possibility.

The relationship between the cultural dissemination of wellness as a way of framing the self and the expansion of addiction discourse is complex. To start with, however, we should establish the rather straightforward temporal coincidence between the two: it was in the 1970s and 1980s that addiction discourse began to suffuse US culture in three discrete, if overlapping, ways.

First, individuals began to identify their own addictions in unprecedented numbers. The most visible face of this development was the explosion of twelve-step and other mutual-help groups for addiction in the 1970s and 1980s. Not only did the member rolls of the existing groups swell rapidly—these decades saw the emergence of many groups devoted to addictions that had never before been claimed. Between 1978 and 1982 alone, four separate "Anonymous" groups for sex addiction were founded, and by the end of the 1980s there were around half a million groups in this country working on addictions involving not just drugs and alcohol but shopping, working, gambling, exercise, and more.[45] One magazine article estimated in 1989 that between twelve and fifteen million Americans were then attending these groups, and a government-funded study found even higher numbers the following year.[46] Meanwhile, specialized periodicals and a burgeoning self-help and pop-psychology literature, sold not only in general bookstores but in the new "recovery stores" founded in the mid-1980s, allowed many others to claim the whole range of addictions.[47]

Second, there emerged in the late 1970s a new academic literature devoted to what we now call behavioral (as opposed to substance) addictions, which gave the new addiction claims in popular culture a scholarly foundation. The journal *Addictive Behaviors* was founded in 1975 to feature research on the full range of addictions, while papers on sex, eating, and gambling addictions appeared with increasing frequency in the more established venues. By the mid-1980s, scholars working to study the commonalities among the various addictions, substance and behavioral, were gathering in national and international conferences and contributing to edited volumes.[48] Although it would take the contributions of neuroscientists in the 1990s to secure a broadened view of addiction as orthodoxy across scholarly fields, the 1980s would be remembered by later scholars as the decade in which the basis for this development was laid.[49]

Third, it was in the 1970s that drug abuse became highly salient as a matter of public and political concern, and this rendered addiction an object of intense interest far beyond those who claimed or studied it. The War on Drugs was declared by Nixon in 1971, marking and driving a surge in popular anxieties about the spread of drug abuse and addiction, whether through the heroin use of Vietnam veterans, the marijuana and alcohol use of suburban teenagers, or the alleged crack use of inner-city youth years later. Rising public concern with addiction was also reflected in other ways. Drug abuse and addiction became ever-more frequent themes in TV sitcoms, for example, as well as in legislative hearings and nightly news reports.[50] And it was in the early 1970s that Gallup began to include drug-related issues in its survey of "national hopes and fears," and these have registered as urgent in polls of public sentiment ever since.[51]

The temporal coincidence of the spread of wellness and the expansion of addiction discourse is no accident, but the sign of a deeper link between them. This link is not strictly causal—neither phenomenon *produces* the other, ex nihilo—and it is not simply a link between two concepts or terms—addiction is not, for instance, the opposite or limit case of wellness. It is instead a kind of kinship: both belong to and elaborate a distinctive imagination of the self, and share an understanding of the relation between the subject's intentional purposes for its existence and the existence that it actually lives. In a word, both discourses articulate the same mode of self-relation. Of course, the two are generically distinct: The one stages and enacts a framework for self-cultivation, while the other examines just one specific condition that may afflict the self. Yet both figure the subject's relation to itself in a twofold way: First, the subject sees itself as the site of an experience that it enacts and must bear, but which is primarily produced by powers and forces that work prior to the conscious interventions of the subject. In wellness, these powers and forces are understood as the effects of fields, environments, and lifestyles in shaping the bodily condition of the self; in addiction, they are (we will see this in detail, momentarily) understood as the array of biological, cultural, psychological, and other forces that incline or outright generate the behavioral tendencies of the self. And second, the subject has an indelibly real capacity to alter its own experience—to cultivate wellness, to reduce addictive behaviors—but this capacity is always mediated by the powers that also and often tacitly shape one's experience; the capacity of the self to remake itself must always pass through and work with those powers, and consists in bending, contesting, or simply comporting with their life-shaping effects.

There is also a historical relationship between the spread of wellness and the expansion of addiction discourse. If neither causes the other, the unfolding of each has nonetheless incited and animated the other's development. In the one direction, the growing specter of addiction spurs the dissemination of wellness practices. It may seem strange to prescribe yoga and jogging as a way to prevent or recover from addiction, yet precisely this has been done now for decades in this country. That is, wellness regimens are often deployed either as part of or even simply *as* addiction treatment—as in the Koch-funded Phoenix gyms intended to combat the opioid epidemic—which is why the Substance Abuse and Mental Health Administration has not only published dozens of pamphlets on wellness but includes a National Wellness Week as part of its National Recovery Month programming efforts.[52] Some have even argued, as in a proposal published by the American Psychological Association, that workplaces should replace drug testing with wellness initiatives as a way of preventing employee addictions.[53] Ardell was right, it would seem, to promote wellness as the means to a "life without crippling dependencies and life-threatening addictions to doctors, drugs, and disease-causing habits."[54]

More consequential, however, has been the other direction of incitement. Here, it is not just that addictions are more likely to be identified as wellness regimens draw more and more attention to what we eat, what we drink, and our bad habits more generally. Further: as wellness has become a widely accepted frame for the human self's experience—once a bizarre watchword of Marin County, wellness is now a section heading in every major US newspaper—addiction has become increasingly legible as a possible and actual threat in that experience. Indeed, in many contemporary accounts of addiction, scholarly and popular, addiction is not just referred to but *explained by* the constitution of the self that we have been studying thus far: that is, we are said to be liable and likely to develop addictions *because* our desire and conduct are formed in the way presumed in wellness. As we have seen, the framework of wellness shows that what we actually want and do are never the direct result of what we intend to want and do; our intention is real, but only one influence, amid the numerous inner and outer influences producing our desire and conduct. In other words, there is always a gap between intention and actuality here, and addiction is the name for the yawning of that gap; it happens, in a sense, *because* the gap is a feature of human existence. The more we see ourselves as bearing such a gap, or more precisely, as being the kinds of creatures who never control what they want or will directly, but who always enact an outcome determined by an array of personal and impersonal forces—the vision of the self actively promoted by and as wellness—the more we see addiction as a ubiquitous possibility of human experience, since we then increasingly see its necessary condition as being in us, in our very constitution as subjects.

To illustrate this last point, let us see how addiction is explained by a selection of recent and especially influential accounts representing three different types of contemporary knowledge about addiction: popular, scientific, and political. In each case, we will encounter the figure of the subject as it is crafted by wellness in an explanatory or generative role in relation to addiction's possibility and reality. We begin with the portrait of the addict in the *Big Book* of Alcoholics Anonymous. First published in 1939, the *Big Book* is nonetheless a contemporary text, in two ways. To start with, its influence on the broader lay imagination of addiction has grown dramatically over the past half century. In 1960, the AA membership numbered one hundred thirty-seven thousand; in the next ten years, this number doubled, and it quadrupled in the following decade. Between 1980 and 1990, the membership grew from just over eight hundred thousand to nearly two million, and spread across the globe.[55] Meanwhile, starting in the 1970s, the principles laid out in the *Big Book* became the model or inspiration for the practices of myriad new non-alcohol-related addiction groups then emerging. There thus arose in this time "a generalized 12-step consciousness," one "founded on a worldview and a set of practices derived from AA" yet exceeding any particular group.[56] This is a worldview charted in the pages of the *Big Book*, and that now circulates much more widely than it could have six decades ago.

Yet it is not just that a formerly esoteric text has now come into the open. Also, the text itself has changed, both materially and in its meaning. The *Book* is composed of two sections, one covering the core principles and early history of the AA movement, and the other a collection of "Personal Stories" meant to illustrate and concretize the principles as they play out in reality. In particular, it is the task of the story section to demonstrate the capaciousness of the religious figures used to elaborate the program of recovery laid out in the first part. According to the *Book*, "each individual, in the personal stories, describes in his own way and from his own point of view the way he established his relationship with God," and diversifying the perspectives from which the stories are delivered has been the explicit purpose of each new revision of the *Book*.[57] Thus, the *Book* has changed in an obvious way since its initial publication: only one of the stories included in the latest edition has survived from the original edition, which featured the accounts of one woman, one agnostic, four others who identified as spiritual but not religious, and twenty-three white male Christians. To be sure, the white-male-Christian view remained dominant even through the third edition, published in 1976, and yet nine of the thirteen stories newly added in that year were explicitly agnostic or atheist or simply elided the role of God in recovery. And in the fourth edition, published in 2001, only eighteen of the forty-two stories feature a Christian God as central, while eleven directly reject that centrality, and the identity features of the story-authors range from white to Black, gay to straight, young to old, American to South Asian, and more. The result of these changes is not only that most of the *Big Book* as it circulates today was absent from the original edition, but that the meaning of the canonical first section too is now different from what it was: less a theory of Christian prodigality and return than an account of *human* tribulation and recovery, a condition "not restricted [by] race, creed, or geography."[58]

So who and what is the addict, according to the *Big Book*? Much of the text is devoted to theorizing "the real alcoholic," whose condition is, at first blush, fully peculiar. "Alcoholics," we learn, are those "who have lost the ability to control [their] drinking."[59] Importantly, this does not mean that the alcoholic has lost control over drinking *tout court*. To begin with, they have the capacity to initiate and even to achieve recovery: "Rarely have we seen a person fail who has thoroughly followed our path. Those who do not recover are people who cannot or will not completely give themselves to this simple program."[60] The powerlessness that the alcoholic avows in the First Step is thus not the inability to stem one's addiction, but to do so without the support of others; hence the AA slogan, "You alone can do it, but you cannot do it alone."[61]

Nor is the alcoholic's loss of control an inability to avoid drinking until and unless they are actively pursuing recovery. In fact, the alcoholic is in general "much like other men" when he "keeps away from drink, as he may do for months and years."[62] What distinguishes the alcoholic is rather the inability to resist a second and third drink, once the first drink has been taken. This is the so-called "allergy" of the alcoholic, an automatic bodily response to alcohol that most do not experience. But here we arrive at a "riddle" at the heart of alcoholism.[63] If the alcoholic can avoid drinking, even for years at a time, and has an allergy that makes alcohol dangerous for him, then why do alcoholics return time and again to drinking despite the danger? (The endless return, and not the allergy as such, is what makes up the condition of alcoholism.) Or, as the *Big Book* puts it, "If hundreds of experiences have shown him that one drink means another with all its attendant suffering and humiliation, why is it he takes that one drink? Why can't he stay on the water wagon? What has become of the common sense and will power that he still sometimes displays with respect to other matters?"[64]

This is where alcoholism finds its roots in the human condition. For the allergy is only a part of the disease: alcoholism is an "illness made up of an allergy plus an obsession," a "disease of a two-fold nature, an allergy of the body and an obsession of the mind."[65] The second part, the obsession, turns out to be fundamental, and it consists in a self-destructive denial of the human condition, a denial that the *Big Book* terms "self-will." According to the fantasy of self-will, each of us *directs* or *stages* our own existence: what we will is what will happen, and our life is like a film that we write, act, and direct by ourselves. Or, as the *Book* makes this point,

> Each person is like an actor who wants to run the whole show; is forever trying to arrange the lights, the ballet, the scenery, and the rest of the players in his own way. If his arrangements would only stay put, if only people would do as he wished, the show would be great [—so he thinks].[66]

Yet invariably, "the show doesn't come off very well," as one might expect whenever an actor tries to administer the entire scene. Such is the delusional state of the alcoholic that keeps him returning to his drug, whether as a direct result of the delusion— thinking that he can will his life in defiance of his allergy—or as an indirect result, that is, as a way of soothing the wounds that he accumulates as he ruins the show of his life in other ways under the spell of his fantasy.

Importantly, this is no delusion of the alcoholic alone. In fact, "most people try to live by self-propulsion," and the *Big Book* provides the examples of "the retired businessman who lolls in the Florida sunshine in the winter complaining of the sad state of the nation; the minister who sighs over the sins of the twentieth century; politicians and reformers who are sure all would be Utopia if the rest of the world would only behave," and more.[67] Each fantasizes that their own purpose could set the world to right, and each is likely to act on this arrogant fantasy, and hence likely to sow chaos in their own life as well as for others. Thus AA founder Bill Wilson writes in *Twelve Steps and Twelve Traditions*, a companion to the *Big Book*, that "the philosophy of self-sufficiency" is "a bone-crushing juggernaut" in modern society. All are ruined by it, not just the alcoholic, and in fact "we who are alcoholics can consider ourselves fortunate indeed," for "each of us has had his own near-fatal encounter with the juggernaut of self-will, and has suffered enough under its weight to be willing to look for something better."[68] "By circumstance rather than by virtue" alcoholics have learned to see the fantasy that sustains their addiction for what it is, and this realization would benefit all, if all were only so lucky.[69]

This is why the "keystone" of the AA recovery program is Step Three: "the decision to turn our will and our lives over to the care of God *as we understood Him*." Simply put, this is a decision to break the illusion of self-will and to lead one's life in accordance with the reality of the human condition, which is to be subjects of an experience arranged by powers beyond our ken and control. Turning over one's will, one does not abdicate responsibility for one's life, but rather vows to act as the "agent" of higher powers that orchestrate the conditions within which life unfolds; it is to vow that "hereafter in this drama of life, God [will] be our Director"; "He is the Principal; we are his Agents." Here, God is the figure for the orchestrating powers, but they are not necessarily Christian or even theistic. In a chapter addressed to "agnostics," the *Big Book* compares the AA figure of God to the natural laws that govern the movement of electrons. "The prosaic steel girder," it explains, "is a mass of electrons whirling around each other at incredible speed. These tiny bodies are governed by precise laws, and these laws hold true throughout the material world." Nothing stranger is said when "the perfectly logical assumption is suggested that underneath . . . life as we see it, there is an All Powerful, Guiding, Creative Intelligence."[70]

Thus, addiction is understood, in the *Big Book*, as proper to the human creature, even as generated by the kind of subject that we are: the conflicts between what one wants for one's life and the actual course that life takes—the essence of an addiction— reflect the structural condition of every human existence, one that is ameliorated only by *abiding* that condition, by bringing one's intentions in line with the higher powers that orchestrate the possibilities of living for each individual. In the *Big Book*, the alcoholic's distinctive allergy is the occasion that brings this con- dition and the way to live it well into view, but it is easy to see how these may be generalized to any other occasion: a susceptibility to work, preaching, or politics, as in the *Book*'s own examples, or to gambling, eating, sex, and shopping—each is the possible site of a ruinous break between what one wills and how one's life un- folds, and hence the possible site of an addiction. For that break is always there, no matter what one is involved in; the question is only whether it will be stretched open, by the delusional acts of self-will, or meliorated, by committing oneself to the prosaic life of the electron, conducted by invisible forces that set the course of its existence.

AA doctrine is often counterposed to the science of addiction, yet the same figure of the self and its explanatory relation to ad- diction has been elaborated in both. Consider the work of the psy- chologist Jim Orford, for example, who is widely recognized as a foundational figure for the scholarly field of behavioral addictions, and whose 1985 *Excessive Appetites* offered the first comprehensive (i.e., non-object-specific) theory of addiction to attract wide no- tice. Like the *Big Book*, Orford's theory presents addiction as "a hu- man potential," as opposed to "a property of those substances and activities" that addictions involve; in other words, addictions grow from within us, from our human constitution, and not out there, from things themselves.[71] Of course, for Orford that constitution is to be understood not in terms of higher powers, but in the idiom of academic psychology. Yet here too the human will be construed as a site where a diverse array of forces produce the life and con- duct of the subject—including, but not privileging, the force of the subject's own agency—and where the nature of this produc- tion allows for the development of a wide variety of addictions.

Drawing especially on the framework of social learning theory, Orford insists that all our behavioral tendencies are "the resultant of opposing forces, some promoting, some restraining."[72] What each of us is likely to do, on any given occasion, is not the spontaneous result of any single cause—whether personal intent or an external stimulus—but rather the actualized form of "the balance struck between inclination and restraint" at that time.[73] The influences that compose this balance are many and multifarious. On the side of promotion, one might find brain adaptations that invest a drug or some other stimulus with tremendous salience within the subject's field of perception, or cognitive expectations of psychological relief or pleasure, or even such forces as peer pressure, cultural glamorization of certain activities, the wish to transgress, and so forth. On the side of restraint, likewise, the relevant forces might include bodily degradation or economic ruin, as well as denunciation from friends and family or social disapprobation, legal restrictions, and personal regret or intent to cease engaging in a problematic form of behavior. Thus, whether and to what extent one is likely to perform a particular act on any given occasion—to drink, to seek sex, to gamble, or even just to do one's work or to buy groceries—is never only compelled or freely willed, but always the result of "the state of the balance sheet" comprising all the forces acting on the self at that time.[74]

This is why, in Orford's view, "the polarity between addiction viewed as voluntary or involuntary, within control or out-of-control, is a false one." Obviously, the addict is not in full control of their behavior; but neither are they fully out of control, at least not in a way that would be distinctive to an addiction. In fact, Orford points out that addictive behavior "is constantly subject to controls in the form of health, legal, economic, and social costs," not to mention the addict's own persistent efforts to give up their addiction.[75] The problem is that these controls are not effective, because an addiction is precisely a condition in which the sum of promoting forces acting on the self "are more than a match for forces of restraint"—that is, so great in magnitude as to render the behavior unresponsive to the application of usual controls.[76] The signature of an addiction is this "reduced responsiveness," well known in "the experience of family members, for example, who become increasingly baffled by repeatedly using to no avail the kinds of informal and usually mild forms of control which are normally effective in influencing other people and in other areas of conduct."[77] It is well known, as well, in the *feeling* of lost control that is partly diagnostic of an addiction. Because the influence of the various forces that promote or restrain behavior "may scarcely be consciously realized," the addict feels as if the normal link between will and conduct has been broken, when in fact the will is active but *outweighed*, along with the other restraining forces, by the huge accumulation of promoting forces on the self.[78]

Conversely, recovery from addiction occurs not when the subject finally reasserts its willful capacity, but when there is "an accumulation of 'losses,' 'costs,' or harm"—that is, of forces of restraint—that can disturb the dominance of the promoting forces and hence render the subject's conduct responsive to the usual controls once again.[79] This is why, Orford argues, so many diverse—indeed contradictory—approaches to therapy, from medical treatment to twelve-step to abstinence-pledge-taking, show such strikingly similar success rates: what matters is less the specific approach they take than their capacity to reinforce the strength of the restraining forces relative to the promoting influences. This can be done by blunting neurological cravings, by the application of social pressures to remain abstinent, or simply by reworking the individual's expectations about the effects of the addictive behavior. All undermine an addiction, because addiction is not finally rooted in a particular kind of cause—biological, psychological, cultural, or anything else—but rather persists so long as there is a gross asymmetry in the self's relevant balance sheet. It follows that the condition of possibility for addiction lies not with any specific etiological factor, but with the fact that the production of the self's conduct takes the form of a balance sheet and is hence susceptible to the imbalance that addiction is. Orford says as much when he insists that "the processes that give rise to strong appetitive attachment [his term for the psychological experience of addiction] are normal ones"—addiction, then, is possible so long as and simply because such processes are normal for the subject.[80]

I want to consider one final instance of the claim that addiction is a liability inherent in the constitution of the self as a site of enactment for a welter of forces, drawn from a discursive vein that is both popular and scientific, where addiction science is explicitly marshaled to shape the relevant political, media, and lay understandings. This is the claim of the National Institute on Drug Abuse, which not only funds 85 percent of all addiction research and thus sets scholarly agendas around the globe, but has also, over the past thirty years, produced a huge number of public-oriented texts and phrases that have been cited or adopted in full by other state agencies, journalists, and politicians at every level. In fact, language crafted by the NIDA is part of every *National Drug Control Strategy* of the last quarter century, and can be found in most national newspaper and magazine articles devoted to addiction and drug abuse in the United States.

The influence of the NIDA has attracted a great deal of criticism from both scholars and practitioners working in the addiction field in recent decades, above all for promoting the brain-disease model of addiction as the exclusive and exhaustive paradigm for studying and treating addiction, but my concern here is not to contest that influence.[81] Rather, it is to show that part of the NIDA's influence has been to disseminate an explanation of addiction that accords with what we have seen in AA and in Orford's theory. Consider how Nora Volkow, director of the NIDA and by far the most prominent spokesperson for the agency, presents the realities of addiction for those seeking to understand the NIDA's theoretical perspective. In 2015, Volkow published two articles that translate this outlook into ordinary language. Noting that "describing addiction as a 'chronic brain disease' is a very theoretical and abstract concept," she boils the concept down to this meaning: "What we mean" is that "a person's brain is no longer able to produce something needed for our functioning and that healthy people take for granted, *free will*." She continues:

All drugs of abuse, whether legal or illegal, cause large surges of dopamine in brain areas crucial for motivating our behavior— both the reward regions . . . as well as prefrontal regions that control our higher functions like judgment, decision making, and self-control over our actions. These brain circuits adapt to these surges by becoming much less sensitive to dopamine, a process called *receptor downregulation*. The result is that ordinary healthy things in our lives—all the pleasurable social and physical behaviors necessary for our survival (which are rewarded by small bursts of dopamine throughout the day)—no longer are enough to motivate a person; the person needs the big surge of dopamine from the drug just to feel temporarily okay . . . and they must continually repeat this, in an endless vicious cycle.[82]

Advanced here is a rather peculiar conception of what constitutes free will. Free will appears, not as a capacity that is *absent* in the addict's condition, but rather as the name for a certain range in motivation that has been reduced for the addict.[83] The addict's brain has become insensitive to all but the most powerful rewards, and so the addict is only motivated by certain stimuli—drugs or some other addictive object. But prior to the addiction, it was not that this same person simply chose what they would do; rather, their free will indexed the *variety* of stimuli by which conduct could be motivated. Moreover, the fall into addiction is not really a fall, but rather the natural result of how human brains "adapt" when powerful rewards are plentiful. Thus, addiction develops, once again, because of the way our conduct happens to be motivated; it is installed, as a possibility, in the constitution of ourselves as acting subjects.

This constitution, and its grounding of addiction's possibility, is even clearer in another article published by Volkow that year, where she likens the addict's condition to life within "a cunningly designed video-game environment" where "challenges to sobriety are around every corner and the person is forced to navigate the environment using a game controller with buttons that are unresponsive or stuck."[84] If addiction represents, as it did in the earlier piece, a *narrowed* repertoire of rewards that can stimulate the subject's conduct, then what is distinctively addictive in this metaphorized condition is the *cunning* of the environment and the *unresponsiveness* of the "gameworld avatar" to the inputs of the player by means of the game controller. The addict may be relieved from this cunning and this unresponsiveness, but not from the broader set of figures constituting the life of the human subject here: first, a split between the experiencing self (avatar) and an intentional self (player) that wants to shape its own experience; and second, the mediation of the self's capacity to shape its own experience by that constitutive split, and by the prior designs and powers within which that experience must unfold.

In this imagination, which runs through Volkow's texts as it does through those of AA and Orford, addiction is essentially human, in two important senses. First, it is a condition that *reflects* the constitution of the subject as an agential subject, namely, as one that bears a split between the self that wills and the self that acts, and that hence always conducts itself only in an indirect and partial way: addiction is, as it were, a permutation of the inevitable detour that links but also separates my intention and my conduct, a detour in which the former always passes by way of the numerous conditions that fight to give rise to the latter. Second, addiction is *rooted* in this constitution. We are liable to addiction because our conduct is produced in the way that it is—that is, produced by the various forces and influences that gather at the site of the subject, whose composite will is actualized as the subject's conduct, often in an unconscious way. This means that the possibility of addiction is tied together with the *truth*—that is, the accepted truth—of this particular constitution of the human. The more our selves assume the form of that constitution—that is, the more we take this constitution as a prism through which to perceive, and as a framework with which to act on, ourselves—the more addiction becomes a present life potential, a real and imminent liability in our experience.

This is why the theory and practice of wellness are so important in inciting and animating the expansion of addiction discourse. Wellness is, as we have seen, precisely a framework—one that is now widely, if surely not always perfectly or exclusively, accepted and assumed by many persons in the United States—within which we view and act on ourselves as creatures embedded in fields of force, conducted by inner and environmental powers that we must abide, bend, or contest. It is a way of figuring and treating ourselves as split, as subjects of our experience, and hence as the kind of creature that addiction discourse reflects and diagnoses. Thus, as wellness has spread as a helpful discourse, disseminating the terms of its mode of self-relation in the United States over the past four decades, it has rendered addiction not just more visible, as we attend to our well-being more vigorously and meticulously, but also more intelligible—we might even say more possible—within the experience of subjects, both in relation to drugs and alcohol and in relation to every other activity and object. The framework of wellness and the specter of addiction incite one another, encourage the other's unfolding, and this reciprocal action expands the circulation of the mode of self-relation that both articulate— its figures, ideals, and precepts for governing the self—as a culturally prevalent truth, or established understanding, of the subject.

At the outset of this chapter, I noted that in recent decades, the expansion of addiction discourse has been read as the symptom of a fatigued and despairing culture, one in which people seem to feel powerless over their lives in nearly every possible domain of experience. In the light of what we have seen, that diagnosis seems to me unsupported, depending as it does on a misreading of what the expanding discourse on addiction actually says. Yet I want to take up the question that animates the diagnosis, which remains, in my view, important and promising: namely, how does the proliferation of addiction as a prism for so many kinds of subjective experience—one that is, moreover, now so often assumed and claimed by individuals themselves—now serve to shape and, in particular, to constrain the ways in which we interpret our own experience? How might it be seen, not simply as a neutral representation of the subject, but as a historically distinctive *bind* that encourages certain ways of seeing and relating to ourselves, while obviating others?

In a text first published in 1992, which remains an important reference in the theoretical literature on addiction, Anthony Giddens poses the question, "Why should addiction have come to be so widely spoken of over the relatively recent period?" and answers that the "proliferation" of addiction discourse is a sign that the coordinating force of tradition has been wholly displaced by the mandate of self-authorship in late-modern Western culture.[85] Giddens writes that ours "is a society in which tradition has more thoroughly been swept away than ever before and in which the reflexive project of self correspondingly assumes an especial importance." In plainer terms, Giddens is describing a social condition in which shared, external rules will no longer be taken as bind-ing upon individual life and conduct; how one lives and what one does are now instead considered to be under the full control of the autonomously deliberating self. Although this new consideration is sometimes celebrated as a form of freedom, it is also, Giddens suggests, a form of obligation: if our lives "are no longer set by pre-existing patterns and habits," this means that "the individual is continually obliged to negotiate life-style options" which then "define who the individual is." Now that the individual is viewed as fully in charge of what they do, a new notion of personal identity, joined with a sense of personal responsibility, emerges. What one does on a daily basis becomes a record of what one has *chosen* to do with and make of one's life—"life-style choices are constitutive of the reflexive narrative of self"—and moral judgments are made about that choice. In particular, Giddens suggests, one's life-style choices must manifest a sense of individuality, demonstrating full and obvious use of one's capacity to craft one's existence. "In a post-traditional order, the narrative of self has in fact to be continually reworked, and life-style practices in line with it, if the individual is to combine personal autonomy with a sense of ontological security"—a sense of freedom and a sense of genuine self.[86]

Addiction thus emerges, in this cultural context, as a failure to meet the requirement of continual and conspicuous self-authorship: it identifies "behaviour counterposed to choice" and hence an abdication of the proper relation one ought to have to one's life and experience. In other words, Giddens considers *addiction* as a pathologizing term, which, when applied, constitutes "a recognition of lack of autonomy that casts a shadow over the competence of the self." It follows that a proliferation of attributed and claimed addictions indicates, first, the extent of the mandate of self-authorship within a culture, and second, the extent to which individuals are found to have failed, or feel themselves to have failed, to meet the terms of that mandate. Giddens writes that "the idea of addiction makes little sense in a traditional culture," where all behavior is *properly* compelled or determined by regulations set over, not by, the self. By contrast, in the late-modern West, every moment in life becomes an opportunity for self-composition, and hence "almost any pattern or habit can become an addiction." "Addictions, then, are a negative index of the degree to which the reflexive project of self moves to centre-stage in late modernity," and of the degree to which that project cannot possibly succeed in a late-capitalist age where individuals are hardly empowered, even as they are expected, to determine their lives by themselves.[87] Yet crucially, it is far from a release from that expectation to have one's conduct tarred as an addiction. In fact, to be labeled as having an addiction is to be further bound by that expectation, insofar as the legitimacy of the expectation is shored up, reinforced, and supplemented by the development of a term that neatly contains, explains, and denigrates instances of conduct that fly in the face of the mandate of self-authorship and self-orchestration.

Curiously, Giddens seems to have read, in contemporary addiction discourse, a premise that it often quite emphatically rejects: that the human subject could *ever* relate to itself as the author is related to a text.[88] Indeed, for Giddens, addiction is the negative product of that premise—the very idea of an addiction, he states, is incoherent without that premise—which figures the subject as single-handedly and fully effectively composing the substance and outcome of its existence. Thus in an essay on AA, for instance, he interprets the twelve steps as an exercise precisely in that kind of self-composition—they train the attending members, he writes, in "a rewriting of the narrative of self."[89] And yet, as we have seen, the possibility of such a writing is considered the ultimate fantasy in the foundational texts of AA; to attempt self-composition is to deny the most basic truth about our own constitution as subjects and our relationship to ourselves. And to live in that fantasy is to guarantee the perpetuation of addiction, not its relief; it is to ensure that, as the *Big Book* put it, the show of one's life will never come off well.

In the place of that fantastic project, the literature of AA—but also contemporary scientific and state literatures on addiction—disseminate a framework for grasping the self's relation to itself in which the self is never the *author* of its existence, but rather the *site* of an existence that it both enacts and observes, one that it may surely partly shape but which is first and foremost shaped by the myriad powers gathered at the site of the subject. This is a self that is never the sole determinant, never the autonomous legislator, of what it wants, does, and pursues, and whose capacity

to affect its own experience is at once real but indirect and un-
privileged, a capacity that is always routed through and contending with the range of inner and outer forces that also strive to
shape that experience. That is, this is a self that is less an author
than an agent of its life, whose dream is not to be sovereign over
itself but to have some say in the crafting of its experience, by
working with and against—by abiding, avoiding, or perhaps even
resisting—the powers, conditions, and designs that set the terms
within which its life unfolds. Such is the self that is structurally
vulnerable to the development of addiction, that is, to a conflict
between conscious purpose and actual will, and that aims to ameliorate this condition through the prism and practices of wellness:
those that allow us to know, or at least to picture, the myriad fields
of force in which we are embedded, and then to alter the effects of
those fields when these become too much for us to bear—not by
heroically transforming those fields or our position within them,
as a director might demand a change of scene, but by rearranging
some part of the environments that conduct our existence, or by
the production of new environments through the cultivation and
stylization of our habits, routines, and techniques.

The point here is not simply to challenge Giddens on the details, but to revise his crucial attempt to answer, by exploring the
expansion of addiction discourse, the question: What effect of
constraint, or tendentious limitation, does the wide circulation of
addiction discourse have on those who receive or accept its terms
and figures as a framework for their experience? That is, what distinct and historically contingent interpretations are we inclined,
rendered more likely, to make of ourselves given the expanded
capacity of addiction discourse to explain how we live and what
we do? For Giddens, the expansion of addiction was a vector of
the larger double bind that holds all late-modern subjects in the
following unlivable position: required to strive for self-authorship,
if not outright self-creation, on the one hand, but condemned to a
ridiculous failure in this striving both by the universal impossibility of individual self-creation, given our nature as socially dependent creatures, and the especial difficulty of self-authorship under
conditions of late, globalized capitalism, on the other. Yet if what
addiction reveals is not actually a *failure* to realize the ideal of self-

authorship, but precisely the general *impossibility* of ever realizing such an ideal, perhaps the bind of an expanded addiction discourse on contemporary self-experience and self-interpretation is rather different from what Giddens described. Perhaps the expanded discourse on addiction constrains us not by extending the fantasy of sovereign individualism but precisely by dealing a death blow to that fantasy, elaborating as the truth of ourselves the fact that we are each, ever and always, conducted by non-subjective forces even as we surely do will for our own existence, being not the masters of ourselves but rather so many sites where vast arrays of powers combine to produce conduct that we enact as agents and vehicles, and never as the sole authors.

I am not here lamenting the death of the sovereign-individualist fantasy; nor do I contest that it is, and always was, a fantasy through and through. My claim is rather that this fantasy does not capture the distinctive bind or constraint circulated and maintained by the expansion of a discourse that increasingly features normalizing constructions of addiction in American late modernity, which is precisely to be figured and formed as a creature whose possible hope for control over its existence is no less individualist, but severely attenuated, indeed finally restricted to navigation of the powers that gather to decide the life of the subject, powers that we may to a certain extent know and contest, but never control—only press against or with using the modest force that is our own conscious will and intention. Perhaps this, then, is the constraint produced on subjects through the circulation of an expansive discourse on addiction, incited and extended by the theory and practice of wellness: a framework of the self that chastens one's ambitions for human control over human existence, and a vision of life itself as suffused by nameless powers that, surrounding us, impinging upon us, condition in large part what we will want, perceive, move toward, and pursue even as we make our own way in and through the world.

Conclusion
Subjects of Accretion

This book has offered an interpretation of some recent and important changes in how addiction and the addict are figured in American science, medicine, and politics. I have argued that across several domains of contemporary knowledge about addiction, we find a development that we can usefully call *normalization*, in which an earlier perspective that cast addiction as a deviation from normal desire, will, and attachment has been displaced or marginalized by a newer understanding of addiction as essentially akin to or continuous with normal experience. Addictive craving, for instance, is today less and less figured as a degraded form of desire, as the primitive hedonism of the animal or the infant, and increasingly construed, in science and the public media that cite it, as a quantitative maximum of desire, extreme in force and intensity yet identical with ordinary wanting in quality and kind. The compulsion of the addict, likewise, is now constructed in our leading diagnostic protocols, treatment methods, and recovery manuals as an intensification of, and not an exception to, how we act in the most normal and healthy scenes of life. And more generally, the figure of dispossession or self-loss once implied by the term addiction is no longer, in the domains that we have studied, considered a special condition of the diagnosed addict. We are all, according to the accounts of addiction examined in this book, exposed and vulnerable to seduction by potent rewarding objects. Indeed, our most quotidian and even most meaningful attachments have their origin, just like our most unusual and painful ones, in the capacity of such objects to powerfully attract us, and to impress their attractive power upon our minds and bodies. In this basic sense, we are all constituted like the addict, and there is no sharp dividing line between the addict and the normal subject. This is not, of course, the sole understanding of addiction now available to us. Yet it is an understanding that is increasingly available to us, and this in a number of widespread and socially influential forms. It has been to reveal this increasing availability, this growing presence, of such an understanding around us that I have developed *normalization* as one prism for making sense of how addiction is thought and constructed in the late-modern United States.

But something more than this presence has been revealed in our study of normalization. In tracing the precise contours and significance of this process, we have been led to articulate several larger cultural developments that are reflected in and bolstered by the normalization of addiction. For, as we have seen, the normalization of addiction is more than a rethinking of addictive craving and compulsion. In every case, it involves a more basic reimagination of human desire, will, and selfhood; hence, the normalization of addiction is also a rethinking of the human subject. Viewed in this perspective, the normalization of addiction appears far from unique or isolated as a cultural development. In fact, it reflects and furthers a number of larger trends in late-modern American society. Chapter 2 revealed how the normalization of addiction through the standardization of behavioral interventions as a treatment modality constructs and governs the subject in a way strikingly consonant with what has been called the postdisciplinary approach to subjects now ascendant in fields such as economic management, criminal justice, education, and public policy. Chapter 3 showed how the de-confessionalization of desire achieved through the scientific normalization of craving, that is, its recasting of the desiring subject as a body whose wanting is pulled by the power of an object and not driven by the upsurge of an inner instinct or soul, has also been achieved through a variety of practices that have become popularized over the last forty years: cognitive behavior therapy, self-tracking, the rating of anything and all. And chapter 4 traced the homology between the self as constructed by the normalization of addiction and that promoted by the discourse of wellness, a homology reflected in the temporal coincidence and mutual incitement between the expansion of addiction discourse and the spread of wellness.

Thus the normalization of addiction appears not as a fully isolated phenomenon but rather as part of a broader set of changes in how the subject is constructed and governed in late-modern American society. In this conclusion, I would like to specify and substantiate this last thesis. How exactly should we understand the broader changes reflected and furthered in the normalization of addiction? Is there a way to synthesize the figure of ourselves that the various developments that we have studied in this book are differently yet perhaps convergently constructing? Who and what are we, if we are increasingly imagined and handled according to the theories and practices that normalize addiction, effect post-disciplinary control over conduct, de-confessionalize desire, and establish the mode of self-relation consecrated in wellness? How do we picture and describe the subject of all these late-modern American cultural developments? To answer these questions in a synthetic or synoptic way, I will move away, in this conclusion, from the more empirically based and specifically focused approach of the main chapters. Instead, I will work at a more abstract level, theorizing the broad and coherent figure of the subject that I see emergent in, and supported by, the full range of late-modern texts, knowledges, and discourses that we have examined.

To enable this work, I want to return one final time to Foucault's own work on the subject, and in particular to his effort to write what he called a history of the modern subject in the West. Foucault was, of course, well aware that there is never one single construction of the subject, one way of figuring and knowing the subject, at a given moment in history. And yet he perceived that there have been certain broad figures or conceptual templates for describing the subject that are especially widely used, and with time tacitly presumed, by many different bodies of knowledge about the human in a given epoch and society. Foucault's own interest was in a figure or template that he considered ubiquitous in modern Western discourses about the human, which rendered the subject, whatever its precise appearance, as a creature whose manifest existence is the expression of a deep-seated and individualized essence or core: a personality, a character, a psyche, or a soul. This broad figure, he argued, informed and found elaboration in the modern Western scientific constructions of the criminal subject and the sexual body, religious and philosophical constructions of the penitent's soul and the moral consciousness, in psychiatric and medical constructions of the individual mind and body, and more. Foucault wanted both to reveal the very ubiquity of the basic figure of the subject as the bearer of a core in Western modernity and to reveal the contingency of this figure, to show its narrowness and peculiarity as a means of depicting the subject, and in doing so to open up the possibility of depicting the subject with other figures and forms. For this, he sought to place the modern figure of the subject in the context of a history, to show its emergence and rise as well as an alternative to its ubiquity.

Foucault's project of a history of the modern subject will support the theoretical effort of this conclusion in two ways. First, it helps to clarify the philosophical status of the broader figure of the subject that I hope to develop. This broader figure cannot stand in for any of the particular constructions of the human that we have surfaced in the various discourses on addiction, therapy, wellness, and more. Nor can it resolve the differences among those particular constructions. The purpose of the figure is rather to reveal the most general and basic *makeup* or *composition* of the human that is accepted and reproduced in each and all of the particular constructions. Foucault's theorization of the subject of essence neither exhausts nor perfectly fits his examples, whether the sexual body as depicted by the modern sexual sciences or the instinctual criminal constructed by modern criminology; and yet, it does capture a broad imagination of the subject that is common to them, and that marks them both as typically modern, as two instances of a broad imagination that became common only in Western modernity. Likewise, the figure that I will be theorizing is meant to draw out what is common and perhaps historically distinctive about the way we are most broadly imagined in all the discourses that this book has studied; it does not capture their full meanings or reduce them to a perfect identity.

Second, Foucault's specific theorization of the modern subject as a being whose life is an expression of its individual essence will help us to define what is distinctive about the subject as it is constructed by the late-modern discourses that we have been studying. Without quite naming it as such, I have already argued that Foucault's figure of the subject of essence captures well, at least in broad outlines, each of the depictions of the human directly challenged or undermined by the cultural developments we have traced in late-modern American society. The addict as bearer of a deformed personality, character, or psyche; the subject whose conduct can be transformed by a disciplining of deep individuality; the subject whose desire is a confession of its inner soul or identity; and the subject whose conscious intent is in direct control of its manifest experience—all of these are constructions that figure the human as a creature that bears in its depths an individual essence or core, and whose life is an expression or elaboration of that essence or core. Insofar as the normalization of addiction, the move to post-disciplinary power, the de-confessionalization of desire, and the spread of wellness as self-relation can be understood as challenges to each of those earlier figures, the new constructions of the human that they yield can be conceived in contrast to the subject of essence. In short, Foucault's modern subject can serve us as a model for what all the cultural developments that we have studied challenge and displace. The new figure of the subject that emerges through the normalization of addiction and its parallel processes can thus be defined as a revision, if not repudiation, of the subject of essence. This will be a figure of the subject that we can consider *late-modern*, both conceptually, since it can be drawn in contrast to the modern subject as Foucault theorized it, and perhaps historically, insofar as it is a figure of the subject that appears increasingly present around us now, more and more instanced in the bodies of knowledge that circulate in our day.

Of course, the question of just how widespread a figure of ourselves that goes beyond the modern subject of essence is, and whether such a figure, if it is widespread, resembles the one that I will be theorizing in this conclusion, can only be answered by further empirical studies. At the end of this conclusion, I will offer tentative sketches of some possible further studies, and make plain my own view that the late-modern subject revealed by the normalization of addiction and its cognate processes is in fact an increasingly important and ubiquitous figure of the subject in late-modern American society. But before going there, let me now reprise Foucault's account of the history of the modern subject, and show how that history might be extended by the figure of the subject that has recurred, in various forms, in this study of the normalization of addiction.

For Foucault, the history of the subject is not a standalone or fundamental narrative. Rather, it is a meta-narrative that serves to draw out the larger significance of the more specified inquiries to which he devoted his writing career: his inquiries into the history of modern psychiatry, the history of the modern sexual sciences, the history of modern punishment practices and criminology, and so forth. The idea of a history of the subject grew from his noticing that a basic and tacit figure of the subject seemed to be presumed in all the various modern bodies of knowledge—or what we can call, for brevity, modern discourses—whose rise he had examined, despite their lack of mutual communication, and despite the different specific terms that these various discourses used to describe their objects (madness, crime, sexuality). This was, as we will see better in a moment, a figure of the subject as the bearer of a personal essence deep within, and for whom any manifest activity or characteristic is an expression or actualization of that latent personal essence. Foucault observed, further, that such a figure was virtually absent, or at least never presumptive, in *early*-modern and medieval discourses on madness, crime, and sex. Thus, the assumption that we are all bearers of personal essences seemed to have become ubiquitous, familiar, and even natural only at a certain point in history. Again, a history of the subject charts how different basic figures of the subject have become ubiquitous, familiar, and natural, accepted in a range of different discourses about the human, in different periods of time. As we discuss the *modern* subject, then, what we will be describing is a figure of ourselves that became widely employed as a framework for human experience starting in the modern, that is, eighteenth and nineteenth, centuries. It will be crucial to keep in mind this more nuanced set of meanings as we now turn to consider one of Foucault's more synoptic accounts of the history of the modern subject, for in his effort to articulate a general framework for his research, Foucault describes this history in rather sweeping terms.

In his lectures at the Collège de France in 1973–74, Foucault is interested in the way that the invention and development of asylum psychiatry in the eighteenth and nineteenth centuries produces a new "apparatus"—that is, a coherent set of observational, descriptive, and therapeutic practices—for constructing the human subject.[1] In other words, the emergence of the asylum as an institution, and of psychiatry as a discourse within that institution, introduces, into the societies where these appear, a novel set of means for describing human beings and imposing the terms of this description on the lives of human beings (i.e., asylum patients). In the third lecture of the series, Foucault steps back from his narration of the history of asylum psychiatry in particular to note that the descriptions and figures of the subject produced by modern psychiatry are deeply consistent with a more general modality of subject-construction that appears across a wide range of intellectual and social domains in the eighteenth and nineteenth centuries. This is what Foucault calls the *disciplinary* modality of subject-construction. Here, *discipline* does not have the specific meaning that it will assume, years later, in *Discipline and Punish* (although its sense here does comprise that later meaning). It does not yet designate an approach to bodily and mental control. Rather, it designates a broad "modality by which political power, power in general, finally reaches the level of bodies and gets a hold on them, taking actions, behaviors, habits, and words into account."[2] For our purposes, the last part of that definition is the most crucial to grasp. Discipline, in these lectures, designates a certain way of *taking hold* of the subject, again not in the sense of taking control, but in the sense of perceiving and producing an account of the subject. It is, as Foucault puts it, a way of *taking actions, behaviors, habits, and words into account,* a way of taking the raw material of subjective experience, as it were, and of turning that material into an account of who and what the subject is. Discipline, in other words, is a modality for *constructing* the subject in discourse. What is more, it is a ubiquitous modality of subject-construction in the modern period. Foucault calls it "the major general form" of discourse about the human subject in the eighteenth century and forward.[3]

But what exactly is this modality? How does it give an account of the subject, and what is distinctive about it? To show this, Foucault places the disciplinary modality in contrast to what he calls the "sovereign" modality of subject-construction. Here again, sovereignty does not denote a specific practice, or method of rule, but rather a way of constructing and "taking hold" of subjects in discourse that Foucault argues was ubiquitous in *early*-modern Western societies. A sovereign discourse—Foucault has in mind the legal, religious, and economic discourses of early-modern France—is distinguished by two features. First, it produces accounts of the subject without tying the figure of the subject to a bodily individuality. When, for instance, the early-modern discourse on legal responsibility produces a figure of the legally culpable subject, or the human insofar as it is capable of legal guilt, it does not produce this as the figure of an *individual*, at least in the sense of a unitary person whose limits are identical with the ends of a singular lifetime and the skin of a singular body. Such a discourse takes into account a set of behaviors, actions, habits, and words, but it does not see these as so many attributes to be tied to an individual who is their source and substance. Foucault writes that in sovereign discourses, "the subject-element is not so much, and we can say that it is almost never, an individual." Instead, actions, behaviors, habits, and words are assigned to or associated with *groups* or *parts* of what we now think of as singular persons or individualities. The subject, in other words, was constructed in the form of "multiplicities situated above physical individuality" or as "fragments or aspects of individuality." So, for instance, one might bear legal responsibility, but not as a singular person, and only "insofar as one is the son of X, bourgeois of this town," or the user of a common road or pasture, or as a composite of bodies in the form of "a family, a community or the inhabitants of a parish." We might go so far as to say that in sovereign discourses, the human *was* always a multiplicity or a fragment of individuality, never an individual, simple and plain. That is, to be described in discourse was to be described *as* a multiplicity or as an aspect of individuality—as a community, or as a son—and not as *this* body which is selfsame across all its various group memberships and partial qualities. In short, the first key characteristic of sovereign discourses on the subject was that they never (or, almost never) rendered the subject as what Foucault calls a "somatic singularity."[4]

The second key characteristic, which follows from the first, is that the account of a human subject given in a sovereign discourse is not permanently tied to any particular somatic instance. In other words, it is not just that descriptions of the subject are incommensurate with individual bodies. Further, they are, as it were, referentially promiscuous. In Foucault's words, "the subject-function moves around and circulates above and below somatic singularities." The description of the subject, and the attributes and capacities of that subject—these are potentially roving, and can pertain to any number of different bodies, or groups, or aspects of bodies. Thus, "I" may speak as the member of a certain parish, but the "I" here only refers to this me, this body, insofar as it is a member of that parish; hence, "I" may as well speak from another body, using a different set of vocal folds; or "I" may well find expression in a chorus of voices at once. There is no discursive appearance or description of the subject that is permanently fixed to any singular body. This is true even of the most apparently singular human subject to appear in sovereign discourses: namely, the literal sovereign, the king. Descriptions of the king may seem to be descriptions of a singular body, and yet, Foucault notes, drawing on Kantorowicz's analysis of the "king's two bodies," actually "the king's body" is never a single body. The subject, king, "must have a kind of permanence" that goes beyond the death of any particular body, "the death of this individual X or Y," if the kingdom is to persist. "More than just his somatic singularity, it must be the solidity of his realm, of his crown," and the fact that another somatic singularity can become king immediately upon the death of X or Y shows that "the king" never really was X or Y, but simply rested upon X or Y momentarily, in a heavy yet incidental way.[5] There is, then, no account of the human in sovereign discourses that is permanently fixed to any particular body; all descriptions of the subject refer promiscuously, attaching to a multiplicity of bodies, circulating continually across, above, and below a variety of somatic singularities.

The emergence of discipline as a modality of subject-construction in discourses such as modern asylum psychiatry represents a sharp departure from the sovereign modality. Against the background of the early-modern sovereign construction of the subject, discipline in general and asylum psychiatry in particular can be interpreted as a "reorganization in depth of the relations between somatic singularity, the subject, and the individual," whose "major effect" is to produce "the historically new element that we call the individual" in high modernity.[6] What characterizes the disciplinary construction of the subject—this new way of taking actions, behaviors, habits, words, and other fragments of experience into account as evidence of who and what the subject is—is its imagination of the subject as *perfectly commensurate with* and *permanently pinned to* an individual body. In Foucault's words, discipline is a modality of subject-construction "by which the subject-function is exactly superimposed and fastened on the somatic singularity."[7] Whenever a disciplinary account of the subject is given, on the basis of certain actions, behaviors, habits, and words that have been performed, that account constructs the subject as an *individual*, that is, as a singular mind or body of which the actions done and words spoken are the personal achievement or expression. What is more, in a disciplinary discourse, the individual becomes not just the agent but also the explanation for the actions and words that are being observed, or accounted for. The individual becomes the *cause* of the experiences that they have or effect; this is why accounts of the subject are permanently tied to individuals, in a disciplinary discourse: what a subject does or says has its root and source within the individual person.

Here is Foucault's most illuminating description of the disciplinary modality of subject-construction. Discipline is a modality of knowledge and interpretation that "fastens the subject-function to the somatic singularity by means of a system of supervision-writing, or by a system of pangraphic panopticism, which behind the somatic singularity projects, as its extension or as its beginning, a core of virtualities, a psyche."[8] To translate this somewhat obscure definition into plainer terms, we might say that discipline is a form of description and observation ("a system of supervision-writing") whose distinctive feature is its projection of a virtual core as the origin and telos of the subject. Discipline, like any other modality of subject-construction, is a way of taking the raw material of human experience into account, and of producing a description or figure of the subject on the basis of such material. But it does so by projecting, or imagining, a core or essence that exists "behind" a body, in a realm of virtuality. This move is crucial, for that core can then serve as the causal source and foundation for the actions, behaviors, habits, and words that need to be accounted for. If each individual body has a personal core or essence *behind* it—in the form of an individual psyche, or a personality, or a soul—then it can serve as an anchor point, as it were, for the life and experience of the subject. It becomes possible to see that the doings and sayings of the subject are *expressions* of an individual person, *emanations from* or *effects of* that individual's unique and underlying core. Thus, who "I" am, or the description of the subject that fits me, can be made fully commensurate with my individual mind and body, for what I do and say cannot be done by any other, since it is causally and ontologically tethered to my personal core. Further, the "I" that I am can become permanently associated with my mind and body, for my core is always in, or rather, *behind* me and my experience, hence prior to and not made by experience; it is my origin and telos—my soul, my character, my psyche. The projection of a virtual core behind each individual somatic singularity is the central move of any disciplinary discourse, which allows any account of the subject to become an exact and permanent description of an individual and renders the subject invariably as an individual.

Again, this abstract description of discipline as a modality of subject-construction is not meant to indicate the existence of some general discourse on the subject in Western modernity. It is, rather, a conceptual framework intended to capture what Foucault discovered to be a common and ascendant modality of subject-construction in modernity, realized only in the concrete and specific discourses that each of his books and lecture courses studied. I have already mentioned that Foucault saw the discourse of modern asylum psychiatry as one example of this disciplinary modality; he saw the figure of the *psyche* emerging in nineteenth-century psychiatric discourse as precisely the stipulation of a personal essence, or virtual core, that was then taken to be a singular and permanent explanation for the manifest actions, behaviors, and words done by the mind and body. But consider, as well, that in *Discipline and Punish*, Foucault is interested in how the novel forms of examination, hierarchical supervision, and spatial arrangement used to govern prisoners in the late eighteenth and nineteenth centuries construct the "soul"—an inner essence that "inhabits [the subject] and brings him to existence"—as the target for judicial and punitive power, as if the criminal acts and interests of the subject are invariably the signs of a deformed or corrupted soul deep within or behind the offending individual's body.[9] Or, in *The History of Sexuality, Volume One*, Foucault takes the modern sexual sciences as, again, a discourse that constructs the sexual subject, for the first time in the late eighteenth and nineteenth centuries, as the bearer of a sexuality, understood as a kind of "saturating" essence that is "everywhere present in [the subject]: at the root of all his actions because it was their insidious and indefinitely active principle," and hence as that "through which each individual must pass in order to have access to his own intelligibility (seeing that it is both the hidden aspect and generative principle of meaning), to the whole of his body (since it is a real and threatened part of it, while symbolically constituting the whole), to his identity (since it joins the force of a drive to the singularity of a history)."[10] And in *Wrong-Doing, Truth-Telling*, Foucault traces the emergence of a new judicial discourse in mid-nineteenth-century France that, in its interrogations of offenders, seeks to know not just the truth of the violation but also the nature of "the criminal subject behind the author of the crime"—the cruel instinct or drive to rebellion "deep down" in the heart of the offender, which gives rise to their deeds.[11] Such are the tangible and separate means by which a disciplinary modality of subject-construction became common, and with time, ubiquitous in the modern Western world.

Just as Foucault used the framework of a history of the subject to reveal both the cultural significance and the specificity of how the subject was being described and imagined in modern psychiatry, criminology, and sexual science, I now want to take the framework that he developed as a means of interpreting the late-modern constructions of the subject that I have analyzed in this study. The various late-modern discourses that we have been examining, I suggest, manifest a distinct and increasingly common way of accounting for the actions, behaviors, habits, and words of the subject in our time, as well as a new reorganization in depth of the relations between individual, subject, and somatic singularity. In other words, these late-modern discourses may be read, I now want to argue, as instances of a new modality of describing and defining the subject—a modality distinguished by its construction of the individual not as the site and expression of a virtual core situated behind and animating the life of the body but as an accretion of life experiences as and in the present life of the body. To clarify this point, I want to stay a bit longer at the conceptual level of the history of the subject, and contrast what I am calling the late-modern modality of subject-construction with both the sovereign and disciplinary modalities. To make this comparison simple, I will illustrate the late-modern modality of subject-construction using the example of the normalizing discourses on addiction, but described in a general way (that is, in a way that could fit any of our specific cases of normalizing discourse, whether the neuroscience of addiction or the theory of drug courts).

It should be clear that the construction of the subject by the various normalizing discourses on addiction sharply differs from what Foucault theorized as the sovereign modality of subject-construction. After all, the understanding of the human constructed by the normalizing discourses on addiction is one that finally pertains to somatic singularities. The descriptions of the subject that are produced within any normalizing discourse on addiction are ultimately characterizations of *this* body or *that* one, in either case an integrated and personalized "I," who is individually an addict or not an addict, whose desire is distributed in certain distinctive ways, who bears motives to pursue these objects and not some others. The subject always appears, or is given an account, in normalizing discourses on addiction, as a figure whose real referent is always an individual, a somatic singularity. It follows that the construction of the subject in the normalizing discourses on addiction *individualizes* the subject in a further sense: not only does it figure a single body; it also provides a means of differentiating one body from another, as well as a framework through which to normatively evaluate that difference. The subject of normalizing addiction discourse is not, then, attached to fragments or agglomerations of bodies; nor does it move from one bodily site to another, circulating above and below somatic singularities.

But neither is the construction of the subject by the normalizing discourses on addiction fully compatible with the disciplinary modality. Within these discourses, the kind of subject that a given body is—an addict, or a non-addict, or a figure in between—is emphatically *not* "exactly fastened" to a somatic singularity, in two senses. As we saw, a disciplinary construction of the subject is fastened to the body through the projection of an ideal or virtual core behind that body, which is the *source* or *cause* of one's life or characteristics as a subject. It is because there exists a destroyed psyche or a corrupted soul behind my body, determining what it is, that I turn out to be an addict, that I desire and act in ways that, at once, class me as an addict-subject and reveal the quality of my psyche or my soul. This means that the construction of the subject in discourse is exhaustively and permanently attached to a somatic singularity—as Foucault put it, the account of oneself as a subject that is given in a disciplinary discourse is not just the description of a present makeup but also of one's "extension," or future, and one's "beginning," or origin. Think again of the modern sciences of sexuality, in which one's sexuality is said to animate and inflect every aspect of one's existence; here, the subject that one is (a heterosexual, or a homosexual, or just simply the kind of creature who will have *an* inner sexuality, whatever it turns out to be) accounts for everything that the body now is, will be, and has been. Whereas in the normalizing discourses on addiction, the construction of a subject as an addict (or otherwise) is never the identification of a psychic depth or core personality. The fact that I am described as an addict or as the bearer of a particular attachment or desire now does not give you insight into my soul or any other virtual essence behind me. It does not give you the generative principle or the comprehensive meaning of me, of my body, or a prediction of any other part of my life and being. In fact, what my addiction tells you is nothing more than that I am constituted like every other subject, and that I have come into repeat contact with those objects whose power of gratification now happens to exert a strong force of attraction on me. The description of desire, in a normalizing addiction discourse, does not project an essence that saturates and comprehends the full life of the body, and that explains, from a position *behind* this body, and *only* this body, why my desire has grown up in me. My desire, thus, will not be read as an expression of my essence, of who I am always and exhaustively; it can only be read as a reflection of some part of what I have done, of what I have encountered, and of where I happen to have been—a reflection of experiences that could have accrued to any other body.

Further, the subject constructed by a normalizing addiction discourse is not *permanently* fastened to any individual body. The point here is not, of course, that one can simply or easily throw off the determination of oneself as an addict (or non-addict) on a whim. To be described as a certain kind of subject is not a casual condition, and indeed either to cultivate a very strong attachment or to recover from a diagnosed addiction, thus changing one's particular status as a subject—both are arduous endeavors, which take time and effort, and which very often fail. And yet, there is no description of the subject in the normalizing discourses on addiction that can be pinned forever to any particular body, that can serve as a timeless and immutable identity for a somatic singularity. This is, again, because the link between descriptions of the subject and the bodies that bear those descriptions is not secured by the projection of a "virtual" reality, behind the phenomenal reality of the body. The identity of the subject is not projected as an ideal substrate of the body. Rather, it is figured as *an accretion on or as the surface of the body*, that is, as a configuration of the body that takes shape over time, and that hardens through the steady repetition of certain experiences of reward and gratification, but that is only and always produced from the material accumulation of bodily encounters with the object world in time. Indeed, the very distinction between *behind* and *on the surface* is abolished. For the phenomenal life of the body, in turn, is no longer figured as an *expression* of a virtual essence, but as the continual accretion of a bodily configuration that, with time, becomes *inclined* or *disposed* in certain ways by the history of its formation. Thus, not just the identity of the subject, but the life of the subject, is figured as accretion, and the subject *is* the set of dispositions built up through the accretion of its living history: who I am is nothing more than the ways in which I tend to desire, think, and act at this moment as a result of what I have enjoyed, encountered, and done in the past, as these collect and compound over time to become the patterns and tendencies that regulate my present actions, behaviors, habits, and words. These dispositions that I am are individual—they serve to describe the bodily life that is now proper to me—but they are not *ideal*—their sources lie not in my soul, but in my history—or *personal*—they are not the expressions of something unique to me, and could just as well be the dispositions of any other subject who encounters what I have encountered. Further, these dispositions that I am may well accrete and accumulate into a radically different shape in my open future. For accretion is a fully material-historical basis and form for the identity and being of the subject: both product and process, it is at once durable in shape yet always in motion, and in this sense ever amenable to assuming a novel form with the continued unfolding of my life experience, inclined by the past but never tethered to a timeless ideality.

Here we have a distinctive modality of subject-construction, a way of figuring the subject as an individual, yet not as the bearer of a timeless essence or identity, and instead as the building up or accretion of a distinctive bodily shape over time, which is never finished. Recall here how we saw the subject of addictive craving being constructed. It is, as always, a matter of observing and evaluating certain manifest phenomena—behaviors, habits, actions, and to a lesser extent in this case, words—and producing an account of who the subject of those behaviors, habits, actions, and words is, of figuring the human in such a way that all these phenomena can be accounted for. Now, we know that when addictive craving is observed, and an individual is constructed as the subject or site of that craving, this can be an enormously consequential act. To be constructed as an addict-subject in this way can be the basis for a medical diagnosis, and lead to administration of medications or behavioral therapies, as well as pernicious social perception and treatment. To be designated as an addict in discourse can even be the basis for a radical restriction of one's civil rights in certain states (Massachusetts, most notably, but also many others) where the law provides for the involuntary commitment of addicts said to be at risk of harming others or themselves. Yet the construction of an individual as a craving, addicted subject will never become a window into the virtual soul that animates the body—craving can never, in the discourses that we have studied, index, as it did in many twentieth-century accounts of addiction, a fractured or collapsed state of the psyche or personality. Rather, it is understood as a building up, an accumulation on the body, or in the nerves, of attachments that have been formed through the repetition and reinforcement of past experiences of gratification: my desire becomes craving not as my immaturity is revealed, but as reward compounds reward and this compounding skews my perception, in a way that is stable but not fixed forever, indeed liable to skewing in new directions. Similarly, we have seen how those motivations which define the addict—the drive to pursue a certain object, and further the drive to do this at the expense of most everything else—are no longer figured as impulses surging forth from or caused by the soul of the subject, but rather, and again, as inclinations instilled in a body by the frequent performance and enjoyment of the act to which one is now driven. And we have seen that behavioral repertoires—habits, mannerisms, obsessions—are not expressions of deep personality flaws but rather patterns set down and ingrained in the body by the cyclical rhythms of daily existence—a fact that at once renders each of us vulnerable to the development of self-destructive conducts and yields a reliable method for changing one's life and comportment, for recovering from an addiction, and for improving one's wellness. In all of these cases, there is a material process of lived history in time that builds on itself and accretes to become a way or style of being: I come to desire, will, and act in ways that are now typical of me, and this typicality allows me to appear in discourse as a certain kind of subject, a certain individual—but this constitution is always both stable and plastic, thick with historical reality yet not ensured by a prior virtuality.

This late-modern construction of the subject further departs from the early-modern and modern modes in its figuration of the body. Although, as noted above, this late-modern subject is unlike the sovereign subject identified with an individual body, it would not be quite right to say that it is fastened to a "somatic singularity" as in the disciplinary modality. For the disciplinary subject, *singularity* describes not just the fact that the body of the subject is individuated—made commensurate with the physical individuality that falls within the bounds of a single skin—but also the fact that the existence of the body falls within certain natural limits determined prior to its lived experience, limits that give the life of the subject a certain integrity and consistency. The modern body expresses or actualizes a virtual core in phenomenal and historical reality, such that this body is a strictly limited form: one whose actual appearance is restricted, from the start and forever, as a set of possible variations on a single theme. The late-modern subject's body is singular in the first sense—it maps onto physical individuality—but not in the second, for it has an openness that is never contained within preset limits. The form that the body takes at one moment will tend to persist, reinforced as it is by the accretion of the past, but this form has no predictive hold on the future, in which further lived experience may have produced the dispositions of this body—hence also the subject that it is—anew. If the modern subject's body was the manifestation of a core potential set down once and for all, we could imagine the body of the late-modern subject as a register and instrument of open, lived history, the corporeal means by which a lifetime of experiences is collected and transposed into the voice and manner of a person, where such transposition is understood as an endless and continuous process: the body as an active relay between experience and expression, rather than the materialization of a fate.

Put another way, the late-modern body is one constituted without a coordinating center. Crucial here is Foucault's claim that disciplinary discourses construct the subject as bearing a "core" behind its phenomenal body, a *single* essence that underwrites not just one way in which the body appears as a subject, but every possible subjective appearance or position that a body can be in the course of its existence. The body, in other words, is figured within the disciplinary modality as housing a basic and central meaning, in the way that a holy text envelops its secret. This is why, Foucault suggests, in the course of modernity, a variety of discourses that construct the subject become substitutable for one another, in a historically novel way: since each account of the subject (as medical patient, as legal offender, as student, and so forth) ultimately assays or indexes the very same center of the body that reveals itself in so many different guises, any one account of the subject could predict or even determine what account that same body will receive in another context. The poorly achieving student, the lazy worker, and the sexual pervert were, then, not just alike but expressions of a single virtual core, and hence always appeared together as various manifestations of the same individual bodies: starting in the eighteenth and nineteenth centuries, Foucault observes, "school classifications are projected, with some modification, but without too much difficulty, into the social-technical hierarchies of the adult world," while "the hierarchism in the disciplinary and military system takes up, while transforming them, the disciplinary hierarchies found in the civil system."[12]

Recall, here, how the addict was figured in many of the twentieth-century reflections on addiction that we have seen. In the scientific and diagnostic constructions of addiction as a sign of psychopathy, in the clinical and political constructions of addiction as a slide into primitivism and mental infancy, in the legal construction of a link between addictive conduct and deeper criminal or antisocial tendencies, the addict was understood to be an exhaustively ruined figure, addiction being the effect, precisely, of a degraded essence or core. Indeed, one is struck to find, not just in political tirades, but in medical-scholarly descriptions of addiction's clinical presentation through much of the twentieth century, a purported deep connection between chronic drug use and sexual disinhibition, irrational thinking, emotional volatility, laziness, criminal tendencies, and more—not simply as statistical correlations, but as the expressions of a common cause.[13] Those links are not fully severed, but are profoundly reimagined, in all the normalizing discourses on addiction that we have examined. For instance, today addiction is surely still associated with criminality, both in fact—the majority of American inmates meet the DSM criteria for substance use disorder[14]—and at the level of discourse, as we saw, for instance, in the theory and institutional design of the drug court. And yet, the association is now most often understood as simply that: association, not deep causal connection. Indeed, even in popular culture the link between addiction and criminality has been relaxed and recast, at least for some addicts: working- or middle-class opioid addicts, especially, are routinely figured in public media as non-criminal, ordinary Americans, if not as exemplary all-Americans. If addicts often appear in court, this is not because of an inner and saturating defect that renders them both drug user and criminal; in fact, there is no single cause at all, only a life lived under certain conditions that made both these developments possible or even likely in ways that cannot easily be generalized across diverse cases. The body is no longer arranged around or by a center; its several aspects coalesce and coincide without merging, adding up to the many ways in which one is presently disposed.

This is not to say, of course, that the late-modern body is labile at every moment, a constant flux of dispositions. The figure of *accretion* is intended to capture how subjective dispositions, tendencies, and habits take on a certain thickness as they are reinforced by a personal history, while keeping in view the full materiality of this reinforcement and what it reinforces. Lived history never sublimates into another form, removed from daily experience, and remains forever open: again, accretion is both product and process, at once—always growing and waning, refining and altering its course and shape. Accretion is a discursive means for constructing the subject, of associating a certain identity with a body, other than those of fastening or anchoring: what secures the association here is perhaps better conceived as a kind of durable adherence, made to stick by the pressures of a past that is heavy yet which continues to shift.

I have drawn this portrait of the subject of accretion, or what we might call a late-modern construction of the subject, on the basis of the kinds of descriptions and interpretations of human experience that we saw, in previous chapters, emerging through the various normalizations of addiction. My claim is that this portrait can help us to comprehend how all the different cases of normalization figure us—not just those of us designated as addicts, but all of us, insofar as the addict is now construed as a normal subject—and what they offer in common as a framework for making sense of our desires, our motivations, and our efforts at self-transformation. I would argue that this portrait can effectively comprehend, as well, some of the crucial constructions of the subject emerging from the several other discourses and practices that we have considered: those of post-disciplinary powers, cognitive behavior therapy, self-tracking, rating, and wellness. And I would wager, in a more speculative way, that it can help us to comprehend how the human subject is being figured, described, and understood in still other domains of contemporary American society and culture. This speculation should, of course, be held in some suspense in the absence of empirical verification. But think, for instance, of how the subject is constructed by the practices of data collection and distribution in our time, which amass and circulate records of what users have browsed, bought, engaged with, or simply left open on their screens as profiles of the kind of user that one is—what products or media one is likely to enjoy, whom or what one is likely to vote for, what passions or rages one is likely to harbor. These profiles are relentlessly identifying and descriptive, and yet they make no claim to know the inner essence of the users that they name; the tendencies and leanings that they capture *are* the subjects to be captured—compiled portfolios of dispositions without depth. Think, also, of how the subject is constructed in the care of mental illness in our day, not in the practices of talk therapy but in the increasingly dominant techniques of psychopharmacology. Today, in the age of Prozac and Ritalin, when one in six Americans takes one or more psychiatric drugs with no illusion that these are silver bullets useful only for the special few who need them, mental pathology and psychic normality are less like character identities (*the* hysteric, *the* neurotic, *the* obsessive-compulsive) than like heart rate or blood pressure— bodily regularities that reflect and respond to the continual influx of substances and impressions as they work on the chemical sites that give rise to varieties of thinking and feeling. Or think of the subject constructed by economic discourses in our day, such as those associated with neoliberalism and finance, wherein the actor of classical liberalism driven dually by competitive fire and natural interest has been displaced by a figure whose identity as worker, producer, and debtor is conditioned, not by inner character or talent, but by a resume of past investments and the market imperatives to which they are now exposed. This survey of possible leads is meant, not as an anticipatory generalization of what I have uncovered in this study of the normalizing discourses on addiction, but rather as a way of formulating an open-ended question that I hope others will be interested in and perhaps pursue: To what extent does the construction of ourselves as subjects of accretion proceed in parallel and find echoes and support elsewhere, beyond the discourses that we have studied, in late-modern American society?

To my mind, the value of answers, even partial answers, to this question would be twofold. First, they would help us to better understand the reasons why so many normalizations of addiction have occurred, and are occurring, in our time. I have been careful not to represent the various larger cultural processes that comprehend and mirror the normalization of addiction as being its direct efficient causes. Yet I do think that there is a relationship of influence among the various cultural processes whose connections I have sought to reveal. My wager is that the more we encounter a certain figure of the subject, even if we encounter it in different forms, in different social venues, and in different languages, the more generally plausible that figure becomes to us—that is, more ordinary, more naturalized, more commonplace. If something like the figure of accretion appears to be the implicit construction of the subject that we encounter in our psychotherapy sessions, or in our wellness practices, or in our digital lives, then we are more prepared, as it were, to accept this figure when it comes to describing our addictions, or even to actively adopt and reproduce this figure if we are in a position to invent and disseminate a new description of addiction, perhaps in the position of scientist, diagnostician, or court official. The dynamic that I am describing is something less than ideological determination and more like a process of gradual familiarization; here, I am affirming and broadening Foucault's own proposition that certain ways of constructing the subject become naturalized, "ingrained in us," by being "relayed through so many different points" to us, that is, by being embodied in a wide array of discourses.[15] Insofar as the normalization of addiction is, at its heart, a construction of the subject as accretion, it is likely to flourish in a cultural context that features many different discourses whose construction of the subject is secured by the figure of accretion; the further description of such a context would serve, in part, to explain the timing and significance of the various normalizations of addiction.

Second, the value of inquiries that seek further instances of a late-modern modality of subject-construction, that is, of discourses constructing the subject using the figure of accretion, would be their capacity to help us better grasp the effect and consequence of the normalizations of addiction. After all, the normalization of addiction is itself one means by which the late-modern modality of subject-construction is being spread and familiarized in our world. The more we hear that addiction is normal, in various strands of scientific, medical, political, and cultural discourse, the more we are exposed to the late-modern figure of accretion that underlies that judgment. The question thus arises: what other discourses in our society, having little to do with addiction but also constructing the subject in a late-modern modality, are legitimated or rendered more plausible in turn as the normalization of addiction proceeds? What new ways of thinking about moral life, or about how to govern unruly or unwanted behavior, or about how to transform oneself, or one's identity, or one's life condition, are indirectly supported by the tacit premise of the normalization of addiction, namely, that the subject can be described, assessed, and treated as if it were simply a material accretion, and with no reference to character, essence, or the soul? And what existential costs, and not only freedoms, may come with the discourses now constructing us, and our lives, through the model of accretion? These are, of course, questions that I have begun to develop by theorizing the links between the normalization of addiction and post-disciplinary power, the de-confessionalization of desire, and the mode of self-relation captured in wellness, but which I hope can be taken much further than I have taken them in this work.

I would like to conclude this text here, at the threshold of future studies, which could take the modality of subject-construction that this book has surfaced as a theoretical prism, both for understanding more richly and deeply the normalization of addiction, and for investigating what Foucault called "the constitution of ourselves" within what may well be a novel chapter in the history of the American subject.

Acknowledgments

I am most grateful to Wendy Brown, whose critical responses to this work enabled all its best observations and ideas. The experience of writing a book in conversation with her has been an extraordinary education, source of joy, and privilege. I am grateful, as well, to Judith Butler, whose reading and questioning of the deepest commitments of this project made revising it a chance for me to think in new ways about discourse, life, and the subject. These two scholars also helped me develop this work in more pragmatic ways; for that too, I am very grateful.

I would also like to thank Jonathan Simon for his advice, conversation, and cheer over several years. His knowledge of the drug policy field, and his recommendation of many useful sources, helped me to find much of the empirical terrain examined in this book. And I thank Stephen K. White for invaluable discussion of my goals for this project at an early stage.

Finally, I would like to thank Karen Merikangas Darling, whose support and advice have helped me to preserve the strengths while repairing the weaknesses of this manuscript, as well as the anonymous reviewers for the press, who have pushed me to make my work more persuasive, more nuanced, and more focused in what it aims to offer to readers.

Earlier versions of chapter 1 and chapter 3 appeared as "Addiction Becomes Normal in the Late Twentieth Century," *History of the Present* 11.1 (2021): 53–79, reprinted with permission of Duke University Press; and "Does Addiction Have a Subject? Desire in Contemporary U.S. Culture," *Journal of Medical Humanities* 42.3 (2021): 435–52. Both essays have been significantly revised for publication here.

Financial support for this work was provided by the University of California, Berkeley, Program in Critical Theory; the University of California Humanities Research Institute; and the Office of the Provost and Dean of the Faculty at Amherst College.

Notes

Introduction

1. A terminological note: in this text, I consistently use the term *addiction* for a phenomenon that has been named in many different ways. I do so, in part, for analytic convenience, but also because the alternative terms that we will encounter (such as *dependence* and *substance use disorder*) were explicitly devised, and are routinely avowed, as specialized ways of naming the condition that is commonly called addiction. The differences among specialized terms are not unimportant, but an umbrella term for the phenomenon that they all address, in different ways, is also scientifically and practically indispensable. Hence, many of the leading scholarly journals that publish research on addiction, variously defined and conceived, feature "addiction" in their titles, while the relevant medical specialty is called "addiction medicine" by groups such as the American Board of Medical Specialties and the American Society of Addiction Medicine, even as addiction is not the standard clinical term. In using "addiction" as the umbrella term in this work, I follow one common and justified, if imperfect, scholarly practice.

2. David Courtwright, "The NIDA Brain Disease Paradigm: History, Resistance, and Spinoffs," *BioSocieties* 5.1 (2010): 140–43.

3. Netherland and Hansen argue that addiction neuroscience, Suboxone, new policy priorities and rhetoric, and what they call "segmented marketing" are the four crucial "technologies" that have carved out a separate way of handling the addictions of American whites. The point that certain cases of normalization pertain especially to white addicts can be extended, at least, to the recasting of national policy rhetoric charted in chapter 1. See Julie Netherland and Helena Hansen, "White Opioids: Pharmaceutical Race and the War on Drugs That Wasn't," *BioSocieties* 12.2 (2017): 217–38; and also Sonia Mendoza, Alexandrea Hatcher, and Helena Hansen, "Race, Stigma, and Addiction," in *The*

Stigma of Addiction: An Essential Guide, ed. Jonathan D. Avery and Joseph J. Avery (Cham, Switzerland: Springer Nature, 2019), 131–52.

4. This characterization holds true nationally, but not necessarily for individual jurisdictions. The racial composition of drug-court clients varies from county to county; in some counties, the client population is almost entirely white, while in others it is mostly Black, or mostly Hispanic. See, for example, Randall T. Brown, "Systematic review of the Impact of Adult Drug-Treatment Courts," *Translational Research* 155.6 (2010): 263–74.

5. Nancy Campbell tells the first story in *Discovering Addiction: The Science and Politics of Substance Abuse Research* (Ann Arbor: University of Michigan Press, 2007). As Campbell puts it, "Neuroscience entered substance abuse research not as a revolution but as a legitimizing force deeply interconnected with behavioral antecedents and with Abraham Wikler's work on conditioning and the role of cues in triggering relapse" (203).

6. Michel Foucault, *Qu'est-ce que la critique? suivi de La culture de soi* (Paris: Vrin, 2015), 128.

7. I adopt this distinction from Judith Butler, *The Psychic Life of Power: Theories in Subjection* (Stanford, CA: Stanford University Press, 1997), 10–11, although I use it in my own way.

8. Michel Foucault, *Subjectivity and Truth: Lectures at the Collège de France, 1980–81* (New York: Picador, 2017), 11.

9. Michel Foucault, *Psychiatric Power: Lectures at the Collège de France, 1973–74* (New York: Picador, 2006), 53.

10. Michel Foucault, *The History of Sexuality, Volume One: An Introduction* (New York: Vintage, 1978), 59.

11. Following Nietzsche, *On the Genealogy of Morals and Ecce Homo*, trans. Walter Kaufmann and R. J. Hollingdale (New York: Vintage, 1967), 21.

Chapter One

1. Scholarly examples of this practice are especially common in the fields of sociology and cultural studies. See, for example, Harry Levine, "The Discovery of Addiction: Changing Conceptions of Habitual Drunkenness in America," *Journal of Studies on Alcohol* 39 (1978): 143–74; Anthony Giddens, "Love, Sex, and Other Addictions," in *The Transformation of Intimacy: Sexuality, Love, and Eroticism in Modern Societies* (Stanford, CA: Stanford University Press, 1992), 65–86; Robin Room, "The Cultural Framing of Addiction," *Janus Head* 6.2 (2003): 221–34; Craig Reinarman, "Addiction as Accomplishment: The Discursive Construction of Disease," *Addiction Research & Theory* 13.4 (2005): 307–20; and Suzanne Fraser et al., "Addiction Stigma and the Biopolitics of Liberal Modernity: A Qualitative Analysis," *International Journal of Drug Policy* 44 (2017): 192–201. The popular version of this practice appears in the discourse on addiction and stigma.

2. Eve Kosofsky Sedgwick, "Epidemics of the Will," in *Tendencies* (Durham, NC: Duke University Press, 1993), 131.

3. William Bennett, *The De-Valuing of America* (New York: Simon & Schuster, 1992), 121, 127, 142.

4. A small selection: Nancy Campbell, *Discovering Addiction: The Science and Politics of Substance Abuse Research* (Ann Arbor: University of Michigan Press, 2007); David Courtwright, "The NIDA Brain Disease Paradigm: History, Resistance, and Spinoffs," *BioSocieties* 5.1 (2010): 137–47; Scott Vrecko, "Birth of a Brain Disease: Science, the State, and Addiction Neuropolitics," *History of the Human Sciences* 23.4 (2010): 52–67; Institute of Medicine, *Pathways of Addiction: Opportunities in Drug Abuse Research* (Washington, DC: National Academy Press, 1996); Institute of Medicine, *Dispelling the Myths about Addiction: Strategies to Increase Understanding and Strengthen Research* (Washington, DC: National Academy Press, 1997).

5. See, for example, Office of National Drug Control Policy, "A Drug Policy for the 21st Century," section on "The Science," *White House*, https://obamawhitehouse.archives.gov/ondcp/drugpolicyreform.

6. David Courtwright, *Dark Paradise: A History of Opiate Addiction in America* (Cambridge, MA: Harvard University Press, 2001), 130–32.

7. Caroline Acker, *Creating the American Junkie: Addiction Research in the Classic Era of Narcotic Control* (Baltimore: Johns Hopkins University Press, 2002), 144.

8. Campbell, *Discovering Addiction*, 16.

9. Lawrence Kolb, *Drug Addiction: A Medical Problem* (Springfield, IL: Thomas, 1962), 38–39. I quote from Kolb's 1962 volume, which reprints several of his early essays from the 1920s along with later contributions.

10. Campbell, *Discovering Addiction*, 16.

11. Courtwright, *Dark Paradise*, 132.

12. Kolb, *Drug Addiction*, 38.

13. Kolb, 39.

14. Kolb, 93.

15. Kolb, 93.

16. Kolb, 85.

17. Campbell, *Discovering Addiction*, 20.

18. Nancy Campbell, "The Conceptual Migration from 'Intoxication of Desire' to 'Disease of Democracy': Addiction, Narcotic Bondage, and North American Modernity," in *The Pharmakon: Concept Figure, Image of Transgression, Poetic Practice*, ed. Hermann Herlinghaus (Memmingen, Germany: Universitätsverlag Winter GmbH Heidelberg, 2018), 101.

19. Sandor Rado, "The Psychoanalysis of Pharmacothymia (Drug Addiction)," *Psychoanalytic Quarterly* 2.1 (1933): 2–5.

20. On Lindesmith's influence, see Darin Weinberg, "Lindesmith on Addiction: A Critical History of a Classic Theory," *Sociological Theory* 15.2 (1997): 150–61; Nancy Campbell, "Addiction," in *Society on the Edge: Social Science and Public Policy in the Postwar United States*, ed. Phillipe Fontaine and Jefferson D. Pooley (New York: Cambridge University Press, 2020), 290–321; and Acker, *Creating the American Junkie*.

21. Alfred Lindesmith, "The Drug Addict as Psychopath," *American Sociological Review* 5.6 (1940): 914; "A Sociological Theory of Drug Addiction," *American Journal of Sociology* 43.4 (1938): 597.

22. Lindesmith, "A Sociological Theory," 599, 606–7.

23. National Institute on Drug Abuse, *Psychodynamics of Drug Dependence* (Washington, DC: US Government Printing Office, 1977), v.

24. National Institute on Drug Abuse, vii.

25. National Institute on Drug Abuse, 20; *Theories on Drug Abuse* (Washington, DC: US Government Printing Office, 1980), xiii.

26. Institute of Medicine, *Pathways*, 14.

27. Institute of Medicine, 36.

28. Institute of Medicine, 87.

29. Institute of Medicine, 48.

30. National Institute on Drug Abuse, *Drugs, Brains, and Behavior: The Science of Addiction*, https://nida.nih.gov/sites/default/files/soa.pdf, 18.

31. Ann Kelley and Kent Berridge, "The Neuroscience of Natural Rewards: Relevance to Addictive Drugs," *Journal of Neuroscience* 22.9 (2002): 3309.

32. E.g., Thomas Insel, "Is Social Attachment an Addictive Disorder?," *Physiology and Behavior* 79 (2003): 351–57; Caroline Davis and Jacqueline Carter, "Compulsive Overeating as an Addiction Disorder: A Review of Theory and Evidence," *Appetite* 53.1 (2009), section on "Food as Drugs," 2; James Burkett and Larry Young, "The Behavioral, Anatomical, and Pharmacological Parallels between Social Attachment, Love, and Addiction," *Psychopharmacology* 224 (2012): 1–26.

33. Isaac Marks, "Behavioural (Non-Chemical) Addictions," *British Journal of Addictions* 85 (1990): 1389.

34. Peter Nathan et al., "History of the Concept of Addiction," *Annual Review of Clinical Psychology* 12 (2016): 34–35.

35. Nathan et al., 35–38; Sean Robinson and Bryon Adinoff, "The Classification of Substance Use Disorders: Historical, Contextual, and Conceptual Considerations," *Behavioral Sciences* 6.3 (2016): 8–11.

36. Mitchell Wilson, "DSM-III and the Transformation of American Psychiatry," *American Journal of Psychiatry* 150.3 (1993): 399–410.

37. American Psychiatric Association, *Diagnostic and Statistical Manual of Mental Disorders: 3rd Edition* (Washington, DC: American Psychiatric Association, 1980), 163.

38. APA, *DSM-III*, 163.

39. Bruce Rounsaville, Robert Spitzer, and Janet Williams, "Proposed Changes in *DSM-III* Substance Use Disorders: Description and Rationale," *American Journal of Psychiatry* 143.4 (1986): 463–68.

40. Rounsaville et al., 465.

41. The background for this work by Edwards and his colleagues was the effort of the World Health Organization, starting in the 1950s, to develop a more clinically sensitive and conceptually consistent set of terms for diagnosing and researching addiction. In 1952, the WHO Expert Committee on Addiction-Producing Drugs proposed a stable definition for addiction, whose meaning was not yet fixed in clinical practice or in the research literature, and in 1957 distinguished between two conditions: drug addiction and drug habituation. In 1964, the Committee proposed yet another term to replace addiction and habituation,

which had "failed in practice to make a clear distinction" and produced "confusion" more generally. This new term was "drug dependence," a "general term" intended to cover the full range of conditions linked with problematic drug use (WHO Expert Committee on Addiction-Producing Drugs, 13th Report, https://apps.who.int/iris/handle/10665/40580). In the 1976 article discussed in the main text and elsewhere, Edwards identifies his work on the "dependence-syndrome" model as an effort to develop the notion of "dependence" that had been introduced but not fully developed by the WHO. For a full account of this history, see James Maddux and David Desmond, "Addiction or Dependence?" *Addiction* 95.5 (2000): 661–65.

42. Griffith Edwards and Milton Gross, "Alcohol Dependence: Provisional Description of a Clinical Syndrome," *British Medical Journal* 1 (1976): 1058.

43. Edwards and Gross, 1060.

44. Griffith Edwards et al., "Nomenclature and Classification of Drug- and Alcohol-Related Problems: A WHO Memorandum," *Bulletin of the World Health Organization* 59.2 (1981): 230.

45. Griffith Edwards, *Matters of Substance: Drugs—and Why Everyone's A User* (New York: Picador, 2004), xxiii–xxiv.

46. Griffith Edwards, "The Trouble with Drink: Why Ideas Matter," *Addiction* 105 (2010): 802. That is, one still either has or does not have a substance use disorder, depending on whether the diagnostician observes a certain minimum number of criteria. Edwards writes "was embraced rapidly by ICD-9 and DSM-III [rather than III-R] . . ."—this is clearly a typo.

47. American Psychiatric Association, *Diagnostic and Statistical Manual of Mental Disorders: Third Edition Revised* (Washington, DC: American Psychiatric Association, 1987), 166–68. The dimensional view of addiction was not only maintained but further affirmed and underscored in DSM-5, as part of a general recognition that for many mental diseases, "from both clinical and research perspectives, there is a need for a more dimensional approach," in contrast to the prevailing "categorial approach." See American Psychiatric Association, *Diagnostic and Statistical Manual of Mental Disorders: Fifth Edition* (Washington, DC: American Psychiatric Association, 2013), 733 and the introduction. For many diseases, however, the DSM-5 maintained a categorial approach to diagnosis; for this story, see Allan Horwitz, *DSM: A History of Psychiatry's Bible* (Baltimore: Johns Hopkins University Press, 2021), chap. 6, "The *DSM-5*'s Failed Revolution," 116–43.

48. Ethan Nadelmann, "Drug Prohibition in the U.S.," in *Crack in America: Demon Drugs and Social Justice*, ed. Craig Reinarman and Harry Levine (Berkeley: University of California Press, 1997), 288–301.

49. Ronald Reagan, "Speech to the Nation on the Campaign against Drug Abuse," September 14, 1986, https://millercenter.org/the-presidency/presidential-speeches/september-14-1986-speech-nation-campaign-against-drug-abuse; "Remarks on the Signing of the Anti-Drug Abuse Act of 1986," October 27, 1986, https://www.reaganlibrary.gov/research/speeches/102786c.

50. Norval Morris, Introduction to *Drugs and Crime: Workshop Proceedings*,

eds. Jeffrey Roth, Michael Tonry, and Norval Morris (Washington, DC: National Research Council), 29.

51. John Goldkamp, "The Origin of the Drug Treatment Court in Miami," in *The Early Drug Courts: Case Studies in Judicial Innovation*, ed. W. Clinton Terry (Thousand Oaks, CA: Sage, 1999), 20.

52. Goldkamp, 20.

53. Peggy Hora et al., "Therapeutic Jurisprudence and the Drug Treatment Court Movement: Revolutionizing the Criminal Justice System's Response to Drug Abuse and Crime in America," *Notre Dame Law Review* 74.2 (1999): 463.

54. Hora et al., 463.

55. Hora et al., 463–64.

56. James Nolan, *Reinventing Justice: The American Drug Court Movement* (Princeton, NJ: Princeton University Press, 2003), especially chap. 8. See also Allison McKim, *Addicted to Rehab: Race, Gender, and Drugs in the Era of Mass Incarceration* (New Brunswick, NJ: Rutgers University Press, 2017); Jennifer Murphy, "Drug Court as Both a Legal and Medical Authority," *Deviant Behavior* 32.3 (2011): 257–91; Kerwin Kaye, "Rehabilitating the 'Drugs Lifestyle': Criminal Justice, Social Control, and the Cultivation of Agency," *Ethnography* 14.2 (2012): 207–32.

57. Hora et al., "Therapeutic Jurisprudence," 482–84.

58. Katharine Sullivan, "Drug Courts Offer a Second Chance," *US Department of Justice*, https://www.ojp.gov/files/archives/blogs/2020/drug-courts -offer-second-chance; Eric Sevigny, "Rethinking Drug Courts against the Backdrop of the Opioid Epidemic," paper presented at the Opioid and Substance Abuse Symposium, April 18, 2018, https://www.uh.edu/hobby/_docs/events /sevignyrethinkingdrugcourtsagainstthebackdropoftheopioidepidemic.pdf; Patti Waldmeir, "'None of These People Ever Gave Up On Me': America's Drug Courts," *Financial Times*, August 23, 2018.

59. See, for instance, Dina Maron, "Drug Courts Appeal to Democrats and Republicans," *Newsweek*, October 6, 2009; Office of National Drug Control Policy, "Drug Courts: A Smart Approach to Criminal Justice," *White House*, https:// obamawhitehouse.archives.gov/ondcp/ondcp-fact-sheets/drug-courts-smart -approach-to-criminal-justice; President's Commission on Combating Drug Addiction and the Opioid Crisis, *Final Report*, 2017, https://www.whitehouse.gov /sites/whitehouse.gov/files/images/Final_Report_Draft_11-1-2017.pdf.

60. John Hagan, *Who Are the Criminals? The Politics of Crime Policy from the Age of Roosevelt to the Age of Reagan* (Princeton, NJ: Princeton University Press, 2003), 16.

61. Alfred Blumstein and Jacqueline Cohen, "Characterizing Criminal Careers," *Science* 237.4818 (1987): 989–91.

62. If this is universally true for nonviolent offenders, in many jurisdictions it is also true for robbers and burglars pending special review. Examples include First Judicial District Adult Drug Court in New Mexico, King County Drug Diversion Court in Washington, Washington County Drug Court in Oregon, and Clayton County Drug Court in Georgia.

63. Richard Nixon, "Remarks on Signing the Comprehensive Drug Abuse

Prevention and Control Act of 1970," https://www.presidency.ucsb.edu
/documents/remarks-signing-the-comprehensive-drug-abuse-prevention-and
-control-act-1970; Richard Nixon, "Remarks at a White House Conference on
Drug Abuse," https://www.presidency.ucsb.edu/documents/remarks-white
-house-conference-drug-abuse.

64. Reagan, "Speech to the Nation"; George H. W. Bush, "Presidential
Address on National Drug Policy," https://www.c-span.org/video/?8921–1
/president-bush-address-national-drug-policy.

65. Bennett, *De-Valuing of America*, 121.

66. Office of National Drug Control Policy, *National Drug Control Strategy*
(Washington, DC: Office of National Drug Control Policy, 1989), 7.

67. Office of National Drug Control Policy, *National Drug Control Strategy*
(Washington, DC: Office of National Drug Control Policy, 2019), 3; Office of
National Drug Control Policy (1989), 8, 94.

68. For example, National Institute on Drug Abuse, "Drug Abuse and Addiction: One of America's Most Challenging Public Health Problems," https://
archives.drugabuse.gov/publications/drug-abuse-addiction-one-americas-most
-challenging-public-health-problems/addiction-chronic-disease; Office of the
Surgeon General, *Facing Addiction in America* (Washington, DC: U.S. Department
of Health and Human Services, 2016), v, 7–16.

69. Barack Obama, "Remarks by the President in Panel Discussion at the
National Prescription Drug Abuse and Heroin Summit," *White House*, March 29,
2016, https://obamawhitehouse.archives.gov/the-press-office/2016/03/29
/remarks-president-panel-discussion-national-prescription-drug-abuse-and.

70. Joseph Treaster, "Ex-Commissioner of New York Named Drug 'Czar,'"
New York Times, April 28, 1993.

71. Office of National Drug Control Policy, *Interim Drug Control Strategy*
(Washington, DC: Office of National Drug Control Policy, 1993), 2.

72. Office of National Drug Control Policy, 4–5.

73. Office of National Drug Control Policy, *National Drug Control Strategy*
(Washington, DC: Office of National Drug Control Policy, 1997), 5.

74. Sally Satel and Scott Lilienfeld, "Addiction and the Brain-Disease Fallacy,"
Frontiers in Psychiatry 4.141 (2014): 4.

75. Karen Kreeger, "Drug Institute Tackles Neurology of Addiction," *Scientist*, August 21, 1995, https://www.the-scientist.com/research/drug-institute
-tackles-neurology-of-addiction-58399.

76. Office of National Drug Control Policy, *National Drug Control Strategy*
(Washington DC: Office of National Drug Control Policy, 2013), iii.

77. Jimmie Reeves and Richard Campbell, *Cracked Coverage: Television News,
the Anti-Cocaine Crusade, and the Reagan Legacy* (Durham, NC: Duke University
Press, 1994).

78. Eric Gibson, "Addiction Lesson in Five Parts: Sick, Blameless," *Wall Street
Journal*, April 3, 1998.

79. Office of National Drug Control Policy, *National Drug Control Strategy*
(Washington, DC: Office of National Drug Control Policy, 2003), 17–18.

80. Office of National Drug Control Policy (2003), 40.

81. Office of National Drug Control Policy, *National Drug Control Strategy* (Washington, DC: Office of National Drug Control Policy, 2009), 15.

82. Drug Policy Alliance, "Critics Call Likely Bush Drug Czar Pick—John Walters . . ." April 24, 2001. http://www.drugpolicy.org/news/2001/04/critics -call-likely-bush-drug-czar-pick-john-walters.

83. John Walters, "Ask the White House," *White House*, December 12, 2008, https://georgewbush-whitehouse.archives.gov/ask/20081212–1.html.

84. Office of National Drug Control Policy, *National Drug Control Strategy* (Washington, DC: Office of National Drug Control Policy, 2005), 36.

85. George W. Bush, "President's Radio Address," *White House*, December 13, 2008, https://georgewbush-whitehouse.archives.gov/news/releases/2008/12 /20081213.html.

86. Obama, "Remarks."

87. A longer argument would be needed to prove this claim; for now, let us simply note that the new public-health framing in political rhetoric is not simply a recognition that addiction is a disease, or even a brain disease, but a new conception of how addiction should be figured as a target for government intervention. In fact, the rhetoric of the War on Drugs (as exemplified, for instance, in the 1989 *National Drug Control Strategy* written under the direction of drug czar William Bennett) was fully compatible with recognition that addiction is a disease; within the War on Drugs rhetoric, such a recognition functioned as further evidence of the fact that addicts were deteriorated creatures (in mind, brain, and body alike) and that drug sellers, who seeded brain disease, among other things, are enemies of society and the state.

88. Centers for Disease Control and Prevention, "Understanding Drug Overdoses and Deaths," https://www.cdc.gov/drugoverdose/epidemic/index .html; Campbell, "Medicalization and Biomedicalization"; Timothy Hickman, "Target America: Visual Culture, Neuroimaging, and the 'Hijacked Brain' Theory of Addiction," *Past & Present* 222.S9 (2014): 207–26.

Chapter Two

1. U.S. Department of Health and Human Services, "National Survey of Substance Abuse Treatment Services," 28–29, available at https://www.samhsa .gov/data/sites/default/files/reports/rpt35313/2020_NSSATS_FINAL.pdf. In fact, medications are only an alternative to behavioral interventions in theory. *In practice*, medication treatment is almost always joined with behavioral interventions, not least because federal regulations require that methadone treatment facilities provide (directly or through a contracted program) "counseling, vocational, education, and other assessment and treatment services," and that physicians refer buprenorphine patients for "appropriate counseling," or behavioral treatment. See the "Federal Opioid Treatment Standards" published in the Public Health chapter of the Code of Federal Regulations, available at https:// www.law.cornell.edu/cfr/text/42/8.12 and the Drug Addiction Treatment Act, available at https://www.congress.gov/bill/106th-congress/house-bill/2634. See also Walter Ling et al., "Comparison of Behavioral Treatment Conditions in Buprenorphine Maintenance," *Addiction* 108 (2013): 1788–98.

2. National Institute on Drug Abuse, *Principles of Drug Addiction Treatment*, 5, available at https://nida.nih.gov/sites/default/files/podat-3rdEd-508.pdf; Office of the Surgeon General, *Facing Addiction in America* (Washington, DC: U.S. Department of Health and Human Services, 2016), 4–14.

3. For an example of the "gold standard" claim, see the following article by then president of the American Medical Association, Barbara L. McAneny, "Landmark Deal on Medication-Assisted Treatment a Model for Nation," *American Medical Association*, January 7, 2019, https://www.ama-assn.org/about /leadership/landmark-deal-medication-assisted-treatment-model-nation; or Office of the Surgeon General, *Facing Addiction in America*, 4–21.

4. Office of the Surgeon General, *Facing Addiction in America*, 4–21.

5. National Institute on Drug Abuse, *Principles of Drug Addiction Treatment*, 5.

6. Kathleen Carroll and Lisa Onken, "Behavioral Therapies for Drug Abuse," *American Journal of Psychiatry* 162.8 (2005): 1452.

7. Carroll and Onken, 1452. Eventually, addiction neuroscience would help to explain and bolster the legitimacy of behavioral interventions as a treatment framework. But the rise of behavioral interventions in the treatment field occurred roughly simultaneously with the rise of neuroscience in the research field and was not an effect of the latter. Initially, the theoretical justification for behavioral interventions was drawn from what (as we saw in chapter 1) was called "behavioral research," and especially from behavioral pharmacology. On the rise of behavioral research in the addiction-science field prior to that of neuroscience, see Nancy Campbell, *Discovering Addiction: The Science and Politics of Substance Abuse Research* (Ann Arbor: University of Michigan Press, 2007), 178–221.

8. Examples of such theorists are cited and discussed in detail in the last section of the chapter.

9. Claire Clark, *The Recovery Revolution: The Battle over Addiction Treatment in the United States* (New York: Columbia University Press, 2017), 187–207.

10. Clark, chap. 6 and conclusion; Meredith Dye et al., "Modified Therapeutic Communities and Adherence to Traditional Elements," *Journal of Psychoactive Drugs* 41.3 (2009): 275–76; and Fernando Perfas, "The Modern Therapeutic Community Model," in *The Opioid Epidemic and the Therapeutic Community Model: An Essential Guide*, ed. Jonathan D. Avery and Christopher A. Kast (Cham, Switzerland: Springer Nature, 2019), 23–44.

11. Perfas, "The Modern Therapeutic Community Model," 27.

12. Robert Hubbard et al., *Drug Abuse Treatment: A National Study of Effectiveness* (Chapel Hill: University of North Carolina Press, 1989), 4. Clark argues that "in 1987, TCs were the most popular treatment type, enrolling more clients than detoxification, maintenance, or multiple-modality treatment centers" (*Recovery Revolution*, 164) but does not provide a source for this claim. I have not been able to verify it independently, and indeed precisely quantifying the number of TCs throughout the 1970s and 1980s is not easy given the existing data. Yet the fact that TCs were a major modality of addiction treatment in those decades is a clear consensus in the scholarly literature on addiction treatment.

13. These are paraphrases of common phrases in the TC treatment literature, actual examples of which appear below.

14. George De Leon, "The Therapeutic Community for Substance Abuse: Perspective and Approach," in *Therapeutic Communities for Addictions: Readings in Theory, Research, and Practice*, ed. George De Leon and James T. Ziegenfuss (Springfield, IL: Thomas, 1986), 7.

15. Daniel Casriel and Grover Amen, *Daytop: Three Addicts and Their Cure* (New York: Hill and Wang, 1971), 147.

16. "The Crack Cocaine Crisis: Joint Hearing before the Select Committee on Narcotics Abuse and Control, House of Representatives and Select Committee on Children, Youth, and Families, House of Representatives," July 15, 1986 (Washington, DC: U.S. Government Printing Office, 1987), 15.

17. George De Leon and James T. Ziegenfuss, preface, *Therapeutic Communities for Addictions*, ix.

18. Reviews by Robert Vaughan Frye in *Journal of Psychoactive Drugs* 19.1 (1987): 109; Victor T. Sturiano in *Psychology of Addictive Behaviors* 2.2 (1988): 96; and Herbert Freudenberger in *Psychotherapy* 24.4 (1987): 830.

19. De Leon, "Therapeutic Community," in *Therapeutic Communities for Addictions*, 17.

20. De Leon, 16, 18.

21. Casriel and Amen, *Daytop*, 136, 143

22. David Kerr, "The Therapeutic Community: A Codified Concept for Training and Upgrading Staff Members Working in a Residential Setting," in *Therapeutic Communities for Addictions*, 60.

23. Martien Kooyman, "The Psychodynamics of Therapeutic Communities for Treatment of Heroin Addicts," in *Therapeutic Communities for Addictions*, 35.

24. From the definition of the TC adopted by the Therapeutic Communities of America in 1979, reproduced in Kerr, "The Therapeutic Community," in *Therapeutic Communities for Addictions*, 57.

25. De Leon, "Therapeutic Community," in *Therapeutic Communities for Addictions*, 9–10.

26. Kooyman, "Psychodynamics," in *Therapeutic Communities for Addictions*, 30.

27. Kooyman, 30–31.

28. Kooyman, 31.

29. Kooyman, 35.

30. Kooyman, 33.

31. Kooyman, 38–39.

32. De Leon, "Therapeutic Community," in *Therapeutic Communities for Addictions*, 7.

33. George De Leon, "The Therapeutic Community: Status and Evolution," *The International Journal of the Addictions* 20.6–7 (1985): 825.

34. Hubbard et al., *Drug Abuse Treatment*, 4.

35. Perfas, "Modern Therapeutic Community Model," 36. See also Dye et al., "Modified Therapeutic Communities"; "TCs Positioning Themselves for New Healthcare Environment," *Alcoholism and Drug Abuse Weekly* 25.8 (2013): 1–3; and National Institute on Drug Abuse, "How Are Therapeutic Communities Adapting to the Current Environment?" available at https://nida.nih.gov/publications/research-reports/therapeutic-communities/how-are-therapeutic

-communities-adapting-to-current-environment. For an investigation of how traditional TC practices do manage to persist in some "modified TC" settings, see Kerwin Kaye, *Enforcing Freedom: Drug Courts, Therapeutic Communities, and the Intimacies of the State* (New York: Columbia University Press, 2019), especially chap. 4.

36. Clark, *Recovery Revolution*, 13.

37. Nancy Reagan, "Drug Q&A for AMA and *Good Morning America*," November 9, 1981, available at https://www.reaganlibrary.gov/public/digitallibrary /smof/speechwriting-speechdrafts/box-435/40-534-5711755-435-020-2018 .pdf, 13; for the larger story of Nancy Reagan's involvement with TCs, see Clark, *Recovery Revolution*, 143–67.

38. Maura Ewing, "The Court System Shouldn't Interrupt the Treatment Process," *Atlantic*, December 16, 2017, https://www.theatlantic.com/politics /archive/2017/12/opioids-massachusetts-supreme-court/548480/.

39. Editorial Board, "If Addiction Is a Disease, Why Is Relapsing a Crime?," *New York Times*, May 29, 2018, https://www.nytimes.com/2018/05/29/opinion /addiction-relapse-prosecutions.html.

40. Deborah Becker, "Court to Rule on Whether Relapse by an Addicted Opioid User Should Be a Crime," *NPR*, October 26, 2017, https://www.npr.org /sections/health-shots/2017/10/26/559541332/court-to-rule-on-whether -relapse-by-an-addicted-opioid-user-should-be-a-crime.

41. "Brief for the Probationer," *Eldred*, 15–16, https://www.ma -appellatecourts.org/docket/SJC-12279.

42. *Commonwealth v. Eldred*, 101 N.E.3d 911 (Mass. 2018), 3, https://law .justia.com/cases/massachusetts/supreme-court/2018/sjc-12279.html.

43. In fact, they also argued that the punishment was unwarranted insofar as the judge should never have assigned a drug-free requirement to someone with addiction, but we will leave that separate argument aside.

44. "Brief for the Probationer," *Eldred*, 2, 32, 37.

45. "Brief for the Probationer," *Eldred*, 15.

46. "Brief for the Probationer," *Eldred*, 6.

47. "Brief for the Probationer," *Eldred*, 15.

48. "Recovery support services" are services that "help to engage and support individuals in treatment," such as "help with navigating systems of care, removing barriers to recovery, staying engaged in the recovery process, and providing a social context for individuals to engage in community living without substance use" (Office of the Surgeon General, *Facing Addiction in America*, 4– 31). Thus, although recovery support services are a crucial adjunct to treatment, they are not, like behavioral interventions and medications, themselves a form of treatment.

49. Nora Volkow, George Koob, and A. Thomas McLellan, "Neurobiologic Advances from the Brain Disease Model of Addiction," *New England Journal of Medicine* 374 (2016): 363. As in Eldred's brief, the article argues for *both* behavioral interventions and medications, but sees the latter as secondary to behavioral interventions: "During treatment, medication can assist in preventing relapse while the brain is healing and normal emotional and decision-making capacities

are being restored"; it is behavioral interventions that promise the primary healing and restoration as they "help to restore balance in brain circuitry that has been affected by drugs" (368).

50. Volkow et al., 364.
51. Volkow et al., 368.
52. Volkow et al., 363.
53. Volkow et al., 366.
54. Volkow et al., 366.
55. As Ruben Baler and Nora Volkow explain this point, in another article devoted to advancing "the paradigm shift needed [for] addressing this disease as a mental health issue": "The decision to act or not to procure a given stimulus will weigh its saliency value in the context of alternative stimuli and as a function of past experiences and of the current internal needs and expectations of the individual" ("Drug Addiction: The Neurobiology of Disrupted Self-Control," *Trends in Molecular Medicine* 12.12 [2006]: 560).
56. Volkow et al., "Neurobiologic Advances," 366; National Institute on Drug Abuse, *Principles of Adolescent Substance Use Disorder Treatment: A Research-Based Guide*, 7, https://nida.nih.gov/sites/default/files/podat-guide-adolescents-508.pdf.
57. Volkow et al., "Neurobiologic Advances," 364.
58. Volkow et al., 366.
59. Volkow et al., 364, 368.
60. For other recent review articles that emphasize these shared strategies of the various behavioral interventions, see Marc Potenza et al., "Neuroscience of Behavioral and Pharmacological Treatments for Addictions," *Neuron* 69 (2011): 696–99; Kathleen Carroll and Bruce J. Rounsaville, "Behavioral Therapies: The Glass Would Be Half Full If Only We Had a Glass," in *Rethinking Substance Abuse: What the Science Shows, and What We Should Do about It*, ed. William Miller and Kathleen Carroll (New York: Guilford, 2006), especially 231–34; Nora Volkow and Marisela Morales, "The Brain on Drugs: From Reward to Addiction," *Cell* 162.4 (2015): 712–25, especially box 5.
61. Volkow et al., "Neurobiologic Advances," 368.
62. National Institute on Drug Abuse, "Contingency Management Interventions/Motivational Incentives," in National Institute on Drug Abuse, *Principles of Effective Drug Addiction Treatment: A Research-Based Guide*, 3rd ed. (Washington, DC: NIDA, 2018), 50–53, https://nida.nih.gov/sites/default/files/675-principles-of-drug-addiction-treatment-a-research-based-guide-third-edition.pdf.
63. National Institute on Drug Abuse, "Community Reinforcement," and "Motivational Enhancement Therapy," in *Principles of Effective Drug Addiction Treatment*, 53–56.
64. National Institute on Drug Abuse, "Cognitive Behavior Therapy," in *Principles of Effective Drug Addiction Treatment*, 49–50.
65. National Institute on Drug Abuse, *Principles of Effective Drug Addiction Treatment*, 6.
66. "What Is LEAD?," *Law Enforcement Assisted Diversion National Support Bureau*, https://www.leadbureau.org/about-lead.

67. For one overview, see Eric Westervelt, "Removing Cops from Behavioral Crisis Calls: 'We Need to Change the Model,'" *NPR*, October 19, 2020, https://www.npr.org/2020/10/19/924146486/removing-cops-from-behavioral-crisis-calls-we-need-to-change-the-model.

68. Michel Foucault, *Discipline and Punish: The Birth of the Prison*, trans. Alan Sheridan (New York: Vintage, 1977).

69. Foucault, 209.

70. Gilles Deleuze, "Postscript on the Societies of Control," *October* 59 (1992): 3–4.

71. Nancy Fraser, "From Discipline to Flexibilization? Rereading Foucault in the Shadow of Globalization," *Constellations* 10.2 (2003): 160.

72. Malcolm Feeley and Jonathan Simon, "The New Penology: Notes on the Emerging Strategy of Corrections and Its Implications," *Criminology* 30.4 (1992): 450.

73. Bernard Harcourt, *Exposed: Desire and Disobedience in the Digital Age* (Cambridge, MA: Harvard University Press, 2015), 17.

74. Deleuze, "Postscript," 7.

75. Fraser, "From Discipline to Flexibilization?," 167–68.

76. Feeley and Simon, "The New Penology," 449, 465.

77. Harcourt, *Exposed*, 89–90.

78. Fraser, "From Discipline to Flexibilization?," 168.

79. Deleuze, "Postscript," 7; Feeley and Simon, "The New Penology," 449–50, my emphasis; Harcourt, *Exposed*, 105.

80. Foucault, *Discipline and Punish*, 138.

81. Foucault, 224–25.

82. Michel Foucault, *Security, Territory, Population: Lectures at the Collège de France, 1977–78* (New York: Picador, 2007), 6.

83. Foucault, 8–9.

84. Grant Farred, "Like Shooting Fish in a Barrel," *Polity* 55.4 (2023, forthcoming).

85. Studies of treatment access disparities by race, gender, class, and geography are numerous, conflicting, and often tentative in their conclusions (because it is so difficult to quantify the complex variables involved). For a sample, see: Fabiola Arbelo Cruz, "Racial Inequities in Treatments of Addictive Disorders," https://medicine.yale.edu/news-article/racial-inequities-in-treatments-of-addictive-disorders/; Nancy Nicosia et al., "Disparities in Criminal Court Referrals to Drug Treatment and Prison for Minority Men," *American Journal of Public Health* 103.6 (2013): e77–e84; National Institute on Drug Abuse, "Sex and Gender Differences in Substance Use Disorder Treatment," https://nida.nih.gov/publications/research-reports/substance-use-in-women/sex-gender-differences-in-substance-use-disorder-treatment; Josh Keller and Adam Pearce, "A Small Indiana County Sends More People to Prison Than San Francisco and Durham, N.C., Combined. Why?" *New York Times*, September 2, 2016, https://www.nytimes.com/2016/09/02/upshot/new-geography-of-prisons.html; Brendan Saloner and Benjamin Lê Cook, "Blacks and Hispanics Are Less Likely Than Whites to Complete Addiction Treatment, Largely Due to Socioeconomic Factors," *Health Affairs* 32.1 (2013): 135–44.

86. I see this thesis as concurrent with (if different in focus from) the views of Julie Netherland, Helena Hansen, and Samuel K. Roberts, who have argued that the emergence of treatment methods that are directed mainly to white addicts does not simply reflect but actively reproduces, and even strengthens, the socially superordinate position of whites in American society. See Julie Netherland and Helena Hansen, "White Opioids: Pharmaceutical Race and the War on Drugs That Wasn't," *BioSocieties* 12.2 (2017), especially 218–20; and Helena Hansen and Samuel K. Roberts, "Two Tiers of Biomedicalization: Methadone, Buprenorphine, and the Racial Politics of Addiction Treatment," in *Critical Perspectives on Addiction*, ed. Julie Netherland (Bingley, UK: Emerald, 2012), especially 97–98.

Chapter Three

1. This construction of addiction as the result of a regression into primitive hedonism emerged in earnest in the early twentieth century in the United States, as Timothy Hickman shows in *The Secret Leprosy of Modern Days: Narcotic Addiction and Cultural Crisis in the United States, 1870–1920* (Amherst: University of Massachusetts Press, 2007) and "Drugs and Race in American Culture: Orientalism in the Turn-of-the-Century Discourse of Narcotic Addiction," *American Studies* 41.1 (2000): 71–91. It persisted throughout the mid-twentieth century, in the form of what Nancy Campbell calls the construction of addiction as a "disorder of desire" in "The Conceptual Migration from 'Intoxication of Desire' to 'Disease of Democracy': Addiction, Narcotic Bondage, and North American Modernity," in *The Pharmakon: Concept Figure, Image of Transgression, Poetic Practice*, ed. Hermann Herlinghaus (Memmingen, Germany: Universitätsverlag Winter GmbH Heidelberg, 2018), 93–123. Examples of this construction can be found in public and scholarly discourse at least through the 1970s and 1980s, as in the book analyzed in the main text below.

2. Donald Ian Macdonald, *Drugs, Drinking, and Adolescents* (Chicago: Year Book Medical Publishers, 1984), 30.

3. Macdonald, 24–27.

4. Macdonald, 25.

5. Macdonald, 98.

6. Macdonald, 97–99.

7. See note 11 below for a clarification of this point.

8. Macdonald makes this point, for example, in *Drugs, Drinking, and Adolescents*, 98.

9. For an account of the stages, see, for instance, George Koob and Nora Volkow, "Neurobiology of Addiction: A Neurocircuitry Analysis," *Lancet Psychiatry* 3.8 (2016), 760–73.

10. Koob and Volkow, 764.

11. There are, of course, competing theories about how dopamine mediates reward in the first stage of addiction, such as the "prediction-error" theory of Wolfram Schultz. For Berridge's own presentation of the incentive-salience theory in the context of a broader debate, see "The Debate over Dopamine's Role

in Reward: The Case for Incentive Salience," *Psychopharmacology* 191 (2007): 391–431. In describing the theory as widely accepted, I do not mean to present it as the only option. Rather, I am pointing to the fact that in many influential presentations of the stages of addiction, the incentive-salience theory is identified either as the primary or exclusive mechanism by which craving initially forms. See, for instance, another widely cited presentation of the stages of addiction by the directors of the National Institute on Alcohol Abuse and Alcoholism and the National Institute on Drug Abuse in Koob and Volkow, "Neurocircuitry of Addiction," *Neuropsychopharmacology* 34 (2010): 217–38, or that provided in World Health Organization, *Neuroscience of Psychoactive Substance Use and Dependence* (Geneva: World Health Organization, 2004), chap. 3. See, as well, the first chapter of the textbook published by the American Society of Addiction Medicine, the leading professional organization for addiction health care providers in the country, which is also authored by Koob and Volkow, and which again presents the incentive-salience theory as the main framework for understanding the initial stage of addiction: "Drug Addiction: The Neurobiology of Motivation Gone Awry," in *The ASAM Principles of Addiction Medicine*, 6th edition, ed. Shannon C. Miller et al. (Philadelphia: Wolters Kluwer, 2019), 3–23.

12. In what follows, I quote mainly from a restatement of the theory published in 2000, which is more succinct than the 1993 article but virtually identical with the earlier piece in its core presentation.

13. Terry Robinson and Kent Berridge, "The Psychology and Neurobiology of Addiction: An Incentive-Sensitization View," *Addiction* 95.S2 (2000): S91.

14. Robinson and Berridge, S92.

15. The converse is also true: some drugs produce strong withdrawal effects but are not addictive, including "some tricyclic antidepressants, anticholinergics, and kappa opioid agonists" (Robinson and Berridge, S92).

16. That is, the behavioral responses that indicate experiences of pleasure still occurred mostly as normal even if the mesolimbic circuits were damaged, and these same responses could not be produced through direct stimulation of the mesolimbic circuits.

17. Robinson and Berridge, "Psychology and Neurobiology of Addiction," S93.

18. Robinson and Berridge, S105.

19. Here we are considering the question: why does anyone take a drug (or engage in some other potentially addictive behavior) to begin with?—a question that is surely important for understanding the full experience of addiction and the development of addictive desire, yet falls outside the specific moment of incentive-salience attribution.

20. Robinson and Berridge, "The Neural Basis of Drug Craving: An Incentive-Sensitization Theory of Addiction," *Brain Research Reviews* 18.3 (1993): 291. It does not matter whether this first stimulation is voluntary or not, which is why desire can be produced by scientists in experimental subjects.

21. Robinson and Berridge, "Psychology and Neurobiology of Addiction," S105.

22. Robinson and Berridge, S109.

23. Robinson and Berridge, S109, S97.

24. "For our purposes craving and 'wanting' differ only in magnitude: craving equals intense 'wanting'" (Robinson and Berridge, "Neural Basis of Drug Craving," 279).

25. Robinson and Berridge, "Psychology and Neurobiology of Addiction," S99.

26. Kent Berridge, "Reward Learning: Reinforcement, Incentives, and Expectations," in *Psychology of Learning and Motivation, Volume 40*, ed. Douglas Medin (Cambridge, MA: Academic Press, 2001), 257; Berridge, "Delight, Desire, and Dread: Generators in the Brain," lecture delivered at Cornell University, May 6, 2016, https://youtu.be/hrf8FlVoR_I.

27. Michel Foucault, *The History of Sexuality, Volume One: An Introduction* (New York: Vintage, 1978), 59–61.

28. Harvey Powelson, quoted in Senate Judiciary Committee, "Marihuana Hashish Epidemic and Its Impact on United States Security" (Washington, DC: US Government Printing Office, 1974), 20–21. For a few relevant examples of the parent-oriented anti-drug surveillance literature, see Marsha Manatt for the National Institute on Drug Abuse, *Parents, Peers, Pot* (Washington, DC: U.S. Department of Health, Education, and Welfare, 1979); Sue Rusche, *How to Form a Families in Action Group in Your Community* (Atlanta, GA: DeKalb Families in Action, 1979); Mitchell Rosenthal and Ira Mothner, *Drugs, Parents, and Children: The Three-Way Connection* (Boston: Houghton Mifflin, 1972).

29. Robinson and Berridge, "Psychology and Neurobiology of Addiction," S100, S105.

30. Here, I provide an abbreviated and tendentious account of psychoanalysis *as it is conceived and rejected* by the CBT theorists that I discuss below. It is not an account of all psychoanalytic practice, although I would suggest that it does capture the broad strokes of the American ego-psychological variant of psychoanalysis that was prevalent at the time that Beck, Ellis, and others staged their interventions into the theory and practice of psychotherapy.

31. Sigmund Freud, *Three Essays on the Theory of Sexuality*, in *The Standard Edition of the Complete Psychological Works of Sigmund Freud, Volume VII*, ed. James Strachey (London: Hogarth, 1953), 239.

32. Paolo Knapp and Aaron Beck, "Cognitive Therapy: Foundations, Conceptual Models, Applications, and Research," *Brazilian Journal of Psychiatry* 30.S2 (2008): S56.

33. Aaron Beck, "Thinking and Depression: II. Theory and Therapy," *Archives of General Psychiatry* 10 (1964): 561–62.

34. Beck, 563.

35. Beck, 563.

36. Beck, 563.

37. Albert Ellis, *Reason and Emotion in Psychotherapy* (Secaucus, NJ: Lyle Stuart, 1975 [1967]), 24–26.

38. Ellis, *Reason and Emotion*, 26–7.

39. "Mobile Fact Sheet," *Pew Research Center*, June 12, 2019, https://www.pewresearch.org/internet/fact-sheet/mobile/.

40. Gina Neff and Dawn Nafus, *Self-Tracking* (Cambridge, MA: MIT Press, 2016), 4.

41. Deborah Lupton, *The Quantified Self* (Cambridge: Polity, 2016), 15. The trend continues to this day. See, for example, James Vincent, "Made to Measure: Why We Can't Stop Quantifying Our Lives," *Guardian*, May 26, 2022, https://www.theguardian.com/news/2022/may/26/measurement-why-we-cant-stop-quantifying-our-lives.

42. Lupton, *Quantified Self*, 12.

43. All quotations of Wolf in the remainder of this section are from his "The Data-Driven Life," *New York Times Magazine*, April 28, 2010.

44. Steven Jonas, "Shelly Jang: Can You See That I Was Falling in Love?" *Quantified Self*, https://quantifiedself.com/blog/shelly-jang-cant-see-falling-love/.

45. Emphasis added.

46. Natasha Dow Schüll, "Self in the Loop: Bits, Patterns, and Pathways in the Quantified Self," in *A Networked Self and Human Augmentics, Artificial Intelligence, Sentience*, ed. Zizi Papacharissi (New York: Routledge, 2019), 33.

47. Some have argued that existing five-star systems are often used *as if* they were binary systems. See Matthew Fisher et al., "Seeing Stars: How the Binary Bias Distorts the Interpretation of Customer Ratings," *Journal of Consumer Research* 45.3 (2018): 471–89.

48. Lauren Goode, "Netflix Is Ditching Five-Star Ratings in Favor of a Thumbs-Up," *Verge*, March 16, 2017.

49. Emphasis added.

50. Kaitlyn Tiffany, "The Tinder Algorithm, Explained," *Vox*, February 7, 2019.

51. Michel Feher, *Rated Agency* (New York: Zone, 2018), 56–57.

52. Feher, *Rated Agency*, 209, 84.

53. Foucault, *History of Sexuality*, 21.

54. Foucault, 59.

55. Foucault, 60.

56. Christopher Bollas, *Meaning and Melancholia: Life in the Age of Bewilderment* (New York: Routledge, 2018), 42–43.

57. Bollas, 64.

58. Joyce McDougall, *Plea for a Measure of Abnormality* (New York: Bunner/Mazel, 1992 [1978]), 213, 215.

59. Bollas, *Meaning and Melancholia*, 42.

Chapter Four

1. In this chapter I use the term *discourse* in a more or less nontechnical sense: as a convenient shorthand for referring to the mass of texts and speech about addiction produced in our society, which has (as will be explained just below) "expanded" considerably over the last forty years.

2. Bruce Alexander and Anton R. F. Schweighofer, "Defining 'Addiction,'" *Canadian Psychology* 29.2 (1988), 151.

3. Robert Kaplan, "Carrot Addiction," *Australian and New Zealand Journal of Psychiatry* 30 (1996): 698–700; Arianne Kouroush et al., "Tanning as a

Behavioral Addiction," *American Journal of Drug and Alcohol Abuse* 36.5 (2010): 284–90.

4. Robert Granfield and Craig Reinarman, "Addiction Is Not *Just* a Brain Disease: Critical Studies of Addiction," in *Expanding Addiction: Critical Essays*, ed. Robert Granfield and Craig Reinarman (New York: Routledge, 2015), 1.

5. Mark Griffiths, "Technological Addictions," *Clinical Psychology Forum* 76 (1995): 14.

6. Steve Sussman et al., "Prevalence of the Addictions: A Problem of the Majority or the Minority?" *Evaluation and the Health Professions* 34.1 (2011): 46.

7. Stanton Peele, *The Diseasing of America: How We Allowed Recovery Zealots and the Addiction Treatment Industry to Convince Us We Are Out of Control* (New York: Jossey-Bass, 1995 [1989]), 232.

8. Anthony Giddens, "Sex, Love, and Other Addictions," in *The Transformation of Intimacy: Sexuality, Love, and Eroticism in Modern Societies* (Stanford, CA: Stanford University Press, 1992); Eve Kosofsky Sedgwick, "Epidemics of the Will," in *Tendencies* (Durham, NC: Duke University Press, 1993).

9. See Maya McGuineas, "Capitalism's Addiction Problem," *Atlantic*, April 2020, https://www.theatlantic.com/magazine/archive/2020/04/capitalisms -addiction-problem/606769/ and David Courtwright, *The Age of Addiction: How Bad Habits Became Big Business* (Cambridge, MA: Harvard University Press, 2019), as well as Adam Alter, *Irresistible: The Rise of Addictive Technology and the Business of Keeping Us Hooked* (New York: Penguin, 2017) and David Kessler, *The End of Overeating: Taking Control of the Insatiable American Appetite* (New York: Rodale, 2009).

10. Michel Foucault, *The Hermeneutics of the Subject: Lectures at the Collège de France, 1981–1982* (New York: Picador, 2005), 10–11.

11. Foucault, 230.

12. Michel Foucault, *The History of Sexuality, Volume Three: The Care of the Self* (New York: Vintage, 1986), 101.

13. For one useful survey, see James William Miller, "Wellness: The History and Development of the Concept," *Spektrum Freizeit* 27.1 (2005): 84–129.

14. On linguists' initial resistance to the term, see Ben Zimmer, "Wellness," *New York Times Magazine*, April 16, 2010, https://www.nytimes.com/2010/04 /18/magazine/18FOB-onlanguage-t.html.

15. Halbert Dunn, "Points of Attack for Raising the Levels of Wellness," *Journal of the National Medical Association* 49.4 (1957): 225; Dunn, "High-Level Wellness for Man and Society," *American Journal of Public Health* 49.6 (1959): 787.

16. Halbert Dunn, "What High-Level Wellness Means," *Canadian Journal of Public Health* 50.11 (1959): 447.

17. Dunn, "Points of Attack," 226.

18. Dunn, "Man and Society," 786.

19. Dunn, "What High-Level Wellness Means," 448.

20. Halbert Dunn, *High-Level Wellness* (Arlington, VA: Beatty, 1961), 17, 14.

21. Dunn, 21.

22. Dunn, "What High-Level Wellness Means," 449.

23. Dunn, *High-Level Wellness*, 191.

24. Dunn, "Points of Attack," 232.

25. Dunn, *High-Level Wellness*, 163.

26. James Miller, "Wellness," 95.

27. Paul Terry, "An Interview with Donald B. Ardell," *American Journal of Health Promotion* 30.2 (2015): TAHP1–7.

28. Donald Ardell, *High-Level Wellness: An Alternative to Doctors, Drugs, and Disease* (Emmaus, PA: Rodale, 1977), 5, 10.

29. Ardell, 6.

30. Ardell, 53.

31. Ardell, 2.

32. Ardell, 7.

33. Ardell, 97.

34. Ardell, 6.

35. Donald Ardell, *14 Days to Wellness: The Easy, Effective and Fun Way to Optimum Health* (Novato, CA: New World Library, 1999 [1985]), 7.

36. Ardell, 14.

37. I am maintaining a stricter and more consistent distinction between *lifestyle* and *environment* than Ardell himself does. On some occasions, Ardell uses lifestyle to refer to the four dimensions of wellness other than environment (the fifth dimension), as in his remark that "physicians who themselves pay little regard to the importance of nutrition, exercise, stress management, and self-responsibility are highly unlikely to promote lifestyle reform to you and me" (*High-Level Wellness*, 50). Thus he often speaks of "lifestyle and environment" rather than lifestyle alone. However, at other times Ardell suggests that environment is a part of lifestyle: he writes, for instance, that "if you combine poor management of stress factors with reckless nutrition, disregard for exercise, dependence on the medical system [i.e., the opposite of self-responsibility], and an adverse environment, you get a lifestyle guaranteed to produce disease and premature death" (*High-Level Wellness*, 135). As I explain in the main text, there is a conceptual difference between environment and the other dimensions of wellness that is important to hold in view, so I stick to the more restrictive usage of lifestyle.

38. Ardell, *High-Level Wellness*, 123.

39. Ardell, 147–48.

40. Ardell, 163.

41. Ardell, 164–165.

42. Daniela Blei, "The False Promises of Wellness Culture," *JSTOR Daily*, January 4, 2017, https://daily.jstor.org/the-false-promises-of-wellness-culture/; Howard Leichter, "'Evil Habits' and 'Personal Choices': Assigning Responsibility for Health in the 20th Century," *Milbank Quarterly* 81.4 (2003): 603–26; Anna Kirkland, "Critical Perspectives on Wellness," *Journal of Health Politics, Policy and Law* 39.5 (2014): 971–88.

43. Andrea Jain, *Selling Yoga: From Counterculture to Pop Culture* (New York: Oxford University Press, 2015); Mark Singleton, *Yoga Body: The Origins of Modern Posture Practice* (New York: Oxford University Press, 2010); Roberta Sassatelli, *Fitness Culture: Gyms and the Commercialisation of Discipline and Fun* (New

York: Palgrave Macmillan, 2010); Shelly McKenzie, *Getting Physical: The Rise of Fitness Culture in America* (Lawrence: University Press of Kansas, 2016); Penelope Latey, "The Pilates Method: History and Philosophy," *Journal of Bodywork and Movement Therapies* 5.4 (2001): 275–82; Weimo Zhu et al., "Clinical Implications of Tai Chi Interventions," *American Journal of Lifestyle Medicine* 4.5 (2010): 418–32; Gyorgy Scrinis, "Functional Foods or Functionally Marketed Foods? A Critique of, and Alternatives to, the Category of 'Functional Foods,'" *Public Health Nutrition* 11.5 (2008): 541–45; R. J. Blendon et al., "Americans' Views on the Use and Regulation of Dietary Supplements," *Archives of Internal Medicine* 161.6 (2001): 805–10; Norman Rosenthal et al., "Seasonal Affective Disorder: A Description of the Syndrome and Preliminary Findings with Light Therapy," *Journal of the American Medical Association Psychiatry* 41.1 (1984): 72–80.

44. David Herzberg, *Happy Pills in America: From Miltown to Prozac* (Baltimore: Johns Hopkins University Press, 2010); Nicolas Rasmussen, *On Speed: The Many Lives of Amphetamine* (New York: New York University Press, 2008).

45. See Klaus Mäkelä et al., *Alcoholics Anonymous as a Mutual-Help Movement: A Study in Eight Societies* (Madison: University of Wisconsin Press, 1996); Marsha Goldsmith, "Proliferating 'Self-Help' Groups Offer Wide Range of Support, Seek Physician Rapport," *Journal of the American Medical Association* 261.17 (1989): 2474–75; Linda Farris Kurtz, "The Self-Help Movement: Review of the Past Decade of Research," *Social Work with Groups* 13.3 (1990): 101–15.

46. Maureen Dowd, "Addiction Chic," *Mademoiselle*, October 1989; Robin Room and Thomas Greenfield, "Alcoholics Anonymous, Other 12-Step Movements, and Psychotherapy in the US Population, 1990," *Addiction* 88.4 (1993): 555–62.

47. Mäkelä et al., *Alcoholics Anonymous*, 224; Stanton Peele, *Diseasing of America*, 115–44; Helen Keane, *What's Wrong with Addiction?* (New York: New York University Press, 2002), 64–68; Robin Room, "'Healing Ourselves and Our Planet': The Emergence and Nature of a Generalized Twelve-Step Consciousness," *Contemporary Drug Problems* 19 (1992): 717–40. See also Giddens, *Transformation of Intimacy*, Sedgwick, *Tendencies*, and Patrick Carnes, *Out of the Shadows: Understanding Sexual Addiction* (Center City, MN: Hazelden, 2001 [1983]) for some examples of the popular literature.

48. Two major conference volumes from this period are William Miller and Nick Heather, eds., *Treating Addictive Behaviors: Processes of Change* (New York: Plenum Press, 1986), and William Miller, ed., *The Addictive Behaviors* (Oxford: Pergamon Press, 1980).

49. See, for example, Mark Griffiths, "Technological Addictions" and Anja Koski-Jännes, "In Search of a Comprehensive Model of Addiction," in *Addiction and Life Course*, ed. Pia Rosenqvist, Jan Blomqvist, Anja Koski-Jännes, and Leif Öjesjö (Stockholm: Nordic Council for Alcohol and Drug Research, 2004), 49–51.

50. See Peele, *Diseasing of America*, for TV examples.

51. David Musto and Pamela Korsmeyer, *The Quest for Drug Control: Politics and Federal Policy in a Period of Increasing Substance Abuse, 1963–1981* (New Haven, CT: Yale University Press, 2002), 39–40.

52. The use of wellness techniques as part of addiction therapy has been made visible in recent articles on the use of running, in particular, as a treatment for addiction. See, for instance, William Shannon, "They Were Addicted to Opioids. Now They're Running the New York Marathon," *New York Times*, November 1, 2018. Perhaps the best-known instance of this phenomenon has been the popularization of Phoenix Gyms, which aim to treat addiction almost entirely through practices ranging from "Crossfit and climbing, to hiking, running, cycling, yoga, and more" (see Phoenix home page at thephoenix.org [accessed March 2020]). These gyms have gained notice thanks to a recent multimillion dollar investment from the Koch brothers (Jennifer Levitz, "Koch-Funded Gyms Help Opioid Addicts Recover," *Wall Street Journal*, September 16, 2016).

53. Joel Bennett and Wayne Lehman, eds., *Preventing Workplace Substance Abuse: Beyond Drug Testing to Wellness* (Washington, DC: American Psychological Association Books, 2003).

54. Ardell, *High-Level Wellness*, 97.

55. Mäkelä et al, *Alcoholics Anonymous*, 26.

56. See Mäkelä et al., 216–27.

57. Alcoholics Anonymous, *Alcoholics Anonymous: The Story of How Many Thousands of Men and Women Have Recovered from Alcoholism* (New York: Alcoholics Anonymous World Services, 2001 [Fourth Edition]), 29. On the purpose of revisions, the *Big Book* states: "All changes made over the years in the Big Book . . . have had the same purpose: to represent the current membership of Alcoholics Anonymous more accurately, and thereby to reach more alcoholics. If you have a drinking problem, we hope that you may pause in reading one of the forty-two personal stories and think: 'Yes, that happened to me'; or, more important, 'Yes, I've felt like that'; or, most important, 'Yes, I believe this program can work for me too'" (xii).

58. Alcoholics Anonymous, 450.

59. Alcoholics Anonymous, 30.

60. Alcoholics Anonymous, 58.

61. This slogan is cited in Linda Farris Kurtz, *Self-Help and Support Groups: A Handbook for Practitioners* (Thousand Oaks, CA: Sage, 1997), 151.

62. Alcoholics Anonymous, *Alcoholics Anonymous*, 22–23.

63. Alcoholics Anonymous, 22.

64. Alcoholics Anonymous, 22.

65. Alcoholics Anonymous, 261; 355.

66. Alcoholics Anonymous, 61.

67. Alcoholics Anonymous, 61–62.

68. Alcoholics Anonymous, *Twelve Steps and Twelve Traditions*, 37–38. Accessed at https://www.aa.org/assets/en_US/en_step3.pdf.

69. A well-known AA slogan goes: "Alcoholics are like everyone else, but more so" (cited in, among many other places, James West, *The Betty Ford Center Book of Answers* [New York: Pocket Books, 1997], 14).

70. Alcoholics Anonymous, *Alcoholics Anonymous*, 48–49.

71. Jim Orford, *Excessive Appetites: A Psychological View of Addictions* (New York: Wiley, 1985), 5.

72. Orford, 158
73. Orford, 210.
74. Orford, 272.
75. Jim Orford, "Addiction Is Not as Puzzling as It Seems," *Behavioral and Brain Sciences* 19 (1996): 591.
76. Orford, *Excessive Appetites*, 279, 239.
77. Orford, 207.
78. Orford, 233, 321.
79. Orford, 272.
80. Jim Orford, "Addiction as Excessive Appetite," *Addiction* 96 (2001): 28.
81. See, for instance, Stanton Peele, "Why We Need to Stop [NIDA director] Nora Volkow from Taking Over the World," https://lifeprocessprogram.com/need-stop-nora-volkow-taking-world/; Marc Lewis, "Why the Disease Definition of Addiction Does Far More Harm Than Good," *Scientific American*, https://blogs.scientificamerican.com/observations/why-the-disease-definition-of-addiction-does-far-more-harm-than-good/; and Sally Satel and Scott O. Lilienfeld, *Brainwashed: The Seductive Appeal of Mindless Neuroscience*. For a historical perspective on these critical debates, see David Courtwright, "The NIDA Brain Disease Paradigm: History, Resistance, and Spinoffs," *BioSocieties* 5.1 (2010): 137–47.
82. Nora Volkow, "Addiction Is a Disease of Free Will," *National Institute on Drug Abuse*, June 12, 2015, https://archives.drugabuse.gov/about-nida/noras-blog/2015/06/addiction-disease-free-will.
83. See chapter 2 for an elaboration of this theory of will.
84. Nora Volkow, "It's Not about Getting High: What Neuroscience Teaches Us about Addiction," *National Council for Behavioral Health*, September 8, 2015, https://www.thenationalcouncil.org/BH365/2015/09/08/getting-high-neuroscience-teaches-us-addiction/.
85. Giddens, *Transformation of Intimacy*, 66.
86. Giddens, 74–75.
87. Giddens, 75–76.
88. He seems, moreover, to maintain a rather high-modern, rather than late-modern, understanding of the relationship between author and text, to borrow the terms of Roland Barthes, "The Death of the Author," in *Image, Music, Text* (London: Fontana, 1977), 145.
89. Giddens, *Transformation of Intimacy*, 103.

Conclusion

1. Michel Foucault, *Psychiatric Power: Lectures at the Collège de France, 1973–74* (New York: Picador, 2006), 13.
2. Foucault, 40.
3. Foucault, 42.
4. Foucault, 44.
5. Foucault, 45.
6. Foucault, 54.

7. Foucault, 55.

8. Foucault, 55.

9. Michel Foucault, *Discipline and Punish: The Birth of the Prison* (New York: Vintage, 1976), 29.

10. Michel Foucault, *The History of Sexuality, Volume One: An Introduction* (New York: Vintage, 1978), 43, 155–56.

11. Michel Foucault, *Wrong-Doing, Truth-Telling: The Function of Avowal in Justice* (Chicago: University of Chicago Press, 2014), 215.

12. Foucault, *Psychiatric Power*, 53.

13. See, for example, Harold Kolansky and William Moore, "Effects of Marihuana on Adolescents and Young Adults," *Journal of the American Medical Association* 216.3 (1971): 486–92; Donald Ian Macdonald, "Drugs, Drinking, Adolescence," *The American Journal of Diseases of Children* [*JAMA Pediatrics*] 138 (1984): 117–25; Gabriel Nahas and Henry Clay Frick II, eds., *Drug Abuse in the Modern World, A Perspective for the Eighties: An International Symposium Held at the College of Physicians and Surgeons of Columbia University* (New York: Pergamon, 1981), especially chapters by Thomas McLellan, George Woody, and Charles O'Brien, Doris Milman, and Harold Voth.

14. *Partnership to End Addiction*, "Substance Abuse and America's Prison Population 2010," https://drugfree.org/reports/behind-bars-ii-substance-abuse-and-americas-prison-population/.

15. Foucault, *History of Sexuality*, 60.

Index

ABC News, 47
abjection, 19–22
abnormality: behavioral interventions
  and, 4, 56–57, 63–64, 70, 75–76,
  80; as fundamental condition, 27;
  measuring desire and, 90, 101;
  normalization and, 21–29, 32;
  permanent distress and, 27; self-
  understanding and, 4, 13
abstinence, 80, 147
Abuse-Dependence distinction, 36
accretion: attachment and, 157–
  58, 170–73; causality and, 167,
  176; clinics and, 175; cognitive
  behavior therapy (CBT) and, 158,
  177; compulsion and, 157–58, 177;
  confessional figure and, 158–59;
  craving and, 157–58, 172–73;
  criminality and, 162, 168, 175–
  76; criminal justice system and,
  158, 169; de-confessionalization
  and, 158–59, 161, 179; desire
  and, 157–61, 169–73, 177, 179;
  diagnosis and, 157, 171–72, 175,
  178; discipline and, 163, 166–68;
  discourse and, 159–79; drugs and,
  169, 175–76; education and, 158;
  emotion and, 175; essence and,

160–62, 167–79; family and, 164;
Foucault and, 159–70, 174–75,
178, 180; habits and, 163–64,
166–69, 172–73, 176; health
and, 157; identity and, 160–61,
168, 171–72, 176–79; impulses
and, 173; individuality and, 161,
164–65, 174; institutions and,
163; knowledge and, 157–62, 166;
language and, 178; legal issues
and, 164, 175; legitimacy and, 179;
media and, 157, 176–77; medicine
and, 157; modality of, 158, 163–
75, 179; modernity and, 160–61,
166–67, 175; moral issues and,
160, 179; motivation and, 4, 173,
177; narratives and, 152–53, 162;
neuroscience and, 169; normalization and, 157–62, 169–71,
175–80; pain and, 158; philosophy and, 160; politics and, 157,
163, 175, 179; post-disciplinary
approach and, 158–59, 177; power
and, 158, 161, 163, 168, 171, 177,
179; prison and, 168; psychiatry
and, 160, 162–63, 166–68, 177;
punishment and, 162–63, 168;
rating and, 158–59; reframing

tracking and, 111; standardization of craving and, 89; television, 14, 46–47, 138; War on Drugs and, 21, 46; wellness and, 129, 132
medication-assisted treatment (MAT), 53, 72–73
medicine: accretion and, 157; addiction and, 5; behavioral interventions and, 53–54, 67, 68, 72, 77, 190n1; buprenorphine, 53; Institute of Medicine and, 30; measuring desire and, 118; naltrexone, 53; normalization and, 19–22, 30; policy and, 51; rating and, 118; reframing self and, 124, 130; Surgeon General and, 53–54
meditation, 129, 134, 136
mental health, 26, 46, 57, 83, 114, 127, 139
metric quantity, 14, 94–95, 105, 112, 114, 117
Miami model, 40–41
military, 9, 21, 48, 175
Miller, James, 132
modality: accretion and, 158, 163–75, 179; attachments and, 1, 25, 55, 91, 170; behavioral interventions and, 53–58, 64, 73, 82–87, 191n12; cognitive behavior therapy (CBT) and, 107; Foucault and, 82–86, 107, 126, 163–70, 175; measuring desire and, 89–91, 107; power of, 13, 55–57, 82–87, 158, 163; reframing self and, 126, 129; research methodology on, 13; treatment and, 1, 13, 53–58, 64, 73, 83, 87, 91, 107, 158, 179
modernity: accretion and, 160–61, 166–67, 175; behavioral interventions and, 82, 86; reframing self and, 153, 155; research methodology and, 15, 17; self-tracking and, 112; Western, 15, 17, 82, 160, 167
moral issues: accretion and, 160, 179; behavioral interventions and, 60–63, 74, 80; collapse of, 20; compass for, 17; drugs and, 20, 29–34, 43, 62–63, 80; ethics, 60, 90–91, 133; Freud and, 107–8; measuring desire and, 90, 92, 108; normalization and, 20, 22, 25, 29, 43–44; psychology and, 12; reframing self and, 135, 152; research methodology and, 12, 17; secular, 135–36; self-understanding and, 12; sex and, 60, 92, 107–8, 160; tainted, 29; wellness and, 135–36
motivation: accretion and, 4, 173, 177; behavioral interventions and, 53, 67, 69–72; competition for, 70–72, 78, 80; flexibility of, 80; inner will and, 74; measuring desire and, 96, 101, 108; normalization and, 28, 50–52; ordinary, 28; policy and, 50–52; range of, 80; reframing self and, 149; rewards and, 70 (*see also* rewards); volition and, 55, 69–70, 74, 79–80; willingness and, 69–70
motivational interviewing, 53, 67
Moyers, Bill, 47

naltrexone, 53
narratives: abjection and, 19–22; behavioral interventions and, 61, 86; Foucault and, 86, 118, 162; measuring desire and, 105, 114, 118; normalization and, 19–23, 46–47, 49; rating and, 118; reframing self and, 152–53, 162; Sedgwick and, 19–21, 125; self-tracking and, 114
Nathan, Peter, 34
National Drug Control Strategy, 44, 47, 68, 148, 190n87
National Institute on Alcohol Abuse and Alcoholism, 68
National Institute on Drug Abuse (NIDA): behavioral interventions and, 53–54, 68; Leshner and, 46; *Pathways to Addiction*, 30–33; policy and, 50; Pollin and, 24; reforming self and, 148; Research Monograph Series, 29–30